Rec'd

284-5369

GIVE
YOURSELF HEALTH

Other books edited by Scott Miners

A Spiritual Approach to Male/Female Relations

GIVE
YOURSELF
HEALTH

THOUGHTS, ATTITUDES & HEALTH

Edited by
SCOTT MINERS

FIRST EDITION

TURNING POINT PRESS

TURNING POINT PRESS
P.O. Box 718, Issaquah, Washington 98027-0718.

Library of Congress Cataloging-in-Publication Data

Miners, Scott
         Give yourself health: thoughts, attitudes and
         health / edited by Scott Miners

         ISBN 0-9625720-0-4

To my father, in whom I saw the power in being human, and to all who think thoughts of health and thus contribute to the wholeness— without fragmentation— of a dynamic and creative world.

Acknowledgements

How does one begin to draw the line between those who have not and those who have, through their lives contributed to the life or project or dreams and goals of another. Doesn't one have to begin with one's kindergarten teacher, parents, and ultimately that mystical realm pre-parents some call God. To begin naming names and praising those whose lives have touched mine, from whom I have learned—and there have been so many—would be to exclude someone, and that I do not do, for it is quite apparent to me how linked we all are. Thus I choose here to acknowledge Life, and those who know me and whose lives have touched mine directly or indirectly also know that in this way I love and acknowledge them for their part in my life, projects and dreams.

Yet, I find myself wanting to name names for those close to me, and from whom I have learned directly or who have helped me with this book, so I will, and if you see your name here, or even if you don't, know I acknowledge you too: Ken, Barb, Cynthia, Craig, Janet, Christopher, Martha for wonders, Jacque and her Z for the inspiration for my chapter and the honor of assisting with *Beyond Common Thought*, which has added immeasurably to my life; Eddie for his popcorn and wonderful humor; Norman and Heidi for computer assistance; George for his time and editing; the genius behind Apple Computers and all those who have made desk-top publishing possible; Rosie, Thunder, their kingdom and the trees outside my window.

Contents

ix

Although numerous methods may be employed by an individual, healing occurs primarily in consciousness.
—George L. Hogben, M.D.

Illness is the result of holding a wrong philosophy, one which permists one to behave foolishly and disharmoniously.
—Henryk Skolimowski, Ph.D.

A healthy consciousness is reflected in a healthy body; the converse connection is equally valid.
—Renée Weber, Ph.D.

It is the use of self, in a loving and compassionate way, which provides us with our most powerful instrument for healing.
—Janet Quinn, Ph.D. R.N.

About the Authors

Deepak Chopra, M.D., trained in India and is a practicing endocrinologist. He is former chief of staff of New England Memorial Hospital in Stoneham, Massachussetts and is founding president of the American Association of Ayurvedic Medicine. He is author of *Quantum Healing* (Bantam, 1989).

Larry Dossey, M.D., is a practitioner of internal medicine with the Dallas Diagnostic Association. He lectures widely, and in 1988 delivered the annual Mahatma Gandhi Memorial Lecture in New Delhi, India. He is the author of *Space, Time and Medicine* (1982), *Beyond Illness* (1984) and *Recovering the Soul: A Scientific and Spiritual Search* (1989).

Blair Justice, Ph.D., a health psychologist and science writer who specializes in behavioral medicine, is the author of the recently-published book *Who Gets Sick: How Beliefs, Moods and Thoughts Affect your Health* (Jeremy Tarcher, Inc., Los Angeles). Dr. Justice is a professor of psychology at the University of Texas School of Public Health in Houston.

Jeanne Segal, Ph.D., is a health psychologist who has been actively involved as a therapist, lecturer and trainer in the emotional and spiritual aspects of catastrophic illness. She has developed an approach to freeing up the emotional blocks associated with fear, numbing and other negative emotions. She is director of Santa Monica-based Project Life, which offers no-cost workshops on the Living Beyond Fear Process to individuals who have tested H.I.V. positive.

Bernie Siegel, M.D., F.A.C.S., is a surgeon in private practice and assistant clinical professor of surgery, Yale University School of Medicine. He is the author of *Love , Medicine and Miracles* and *Peace, Love and Healing* (both Harper & Row). The article "Spiritual Aspects of the Healing Arts" was first published in *The American Theosophist*, Vol 72, No. 5, 1984.

Complete health and awakening are really the same.

—Tarthang Tulku

Introduction:
Health and The Mystical

Scott Miners

T HE SEVEN BLIND MEN AND THE ELEPHANT story is quite famous, and well it should be. The story depicts the blind men each touching a different part of the elephant and proclaiming authoritatively their view of the true nature of the animal. I would like to tell the elephant story with a small new twist.

This idea first occured to me when I was in graduate school studying counseling psychology. The many psychological theories we have today are wonderful in their descriptions of human nature, and I thought one day, if someone were to put them all together, we may have the whole elephant. Well, that notion approaches the truth, but, given the dynamic and infinite nature of human growth and discovery, it doesn't seem likely that anyone will ever describe it all, at least not in words. Be that as it

---

may, perhaps a story, like myth, can help point the way beyond the limits we sometimes erect around our worldviews with words.

In the spirit of exploration then, here is the new elephant story with some different blind men: One day a biologist, a chemist, a physicist, an astronomer, an historian, a preacher, a psychologist and a mystic, all fledglings in their respective trades, were standing together discussing their differing perspectives about life. Differ as they may, they all had at least one thing in common—they had temporary animal amnesia, which is a rare disease; it renders one unable to recall anything about animals at all, although all other brain functions remain quite normal. During their lively discussion they noticed an elephant in front of them. They had a curious feeling about what the thing might be, but couldn't quite make it out, so they ventured forth to analyze what they called "the beast."

The biologist took a cell culture and pronounced the beast to be made up of some fundamental structures common to all known life on Earth. The chemist analyzed the same culture and made a similar announcement, with a bit of a "refinement." The physicist drew forth his pocket electron microsope, analyzed the tissue and said, "Ah, I see something, but I cannot determine whether it is a particle or a wave." The astronomer then spoke and said, "Seemingly the thing is from this planet, but much more analysis is needed of a new quasar that has just been discovered before we can discern the true origin of this enormous beast." The historian held, from his knowledge of archaeology, that the beast must indeed be related to a certain warrior tribe on another continent, but, since his information was based upon the story of another ("his" story), he had no further comment. The preacher said that the beast was simply sent by God to remind us all that we need to repent for our sins and send money to his church, which actions could effectively be completed by taking the latter one alone. The psychologist, a fundamental behaviorist, jabbed the beast in the hindquarter, whereon it reared up and galloped off into the distance. "Ah," he said, "it is averse to pain." Thereon he proposed a theory: "If something responds to a stimulus, it is not only alive, but it may be possible to condition it to do anything we like." The mystic watched as the beast ran away. All awaited his answer, since he alone remained silent.

He thought to himself, "These learned men have all spoken so eloquently, but I do not think I have a greater understanding of the identity of this beast than I did before they spoke. In fact, I feel a little confused. As I observed the animal, I noticed a feeling of awe about its presence, as I did about my friends, and I felt fine with that view. Now, however, I need to evaluate the findings of my cohorts. Still, I do feel a sense of wonder about the beast."

The others urged him to speak saying "what is your opinion mystic, you have not yet spoken?" With profound longing in his soul to understand, but knowing his words were inadequate, he said only, "You have all identified aspects of this beast, but truly the being is not separate from the Source from which it came." With that the members of the group departed mumbling to themselves, "What did you expect, he has always been a dreamer."

The mystic, alone, sat in contemplation awhile

beneath the shade of a tree. He spoke to his inner Self saying, "I want to know. I know all knowledge exists in the Great Mind." As he thus desired and contemplated, a thought flashed forth from his mind, the synapses in his brain responded and he exclaimed, "Ah, the beast; it was an elephant!"

The mystic thus found, through his desire—a key element—and his listening for a response in contemplation, that an understanding is gained.

It is much the same in healing. The mystic (everyone of us) listened for his answer—but he *asked* the question. Larry Dossey, M.D. speaks to this passive/active role in healing in his article "The Hidden Dimensions of Health" that follows. He writes of Era III medicine where there is acknowledgement of the Great Mind, or divine aspect of the Universe as the healer, the wholeness that can bring healing.

A health issue often raised is, "Do we want healing, or do we want an illness?" In the space/ simultaneity of time continuum of the mystical mind we have to ask, " What is it that we want to get ourselves to live and do in life and how have we done that?" Blair Justice, Ph.D., writes in his article "Can We Decide when to Get Sick and When Not To?" about how talking to self, to our bodies, just as the mystic spoke to his inner Self, can bring health. Indeed, can thoughts heal the body because thoughts created its need to be healed?

How can we know? Knowing in the "mystical" sense is equated with an expanded sense of awareness.

———

Those in the elephant story each had a belief system through which they analyzed the elephant. Their thoughts and attitudes influenced the way they perceived the beast. Isn't that very much what we do with our lives? We could say that our lives dwell within our belief systems. The mystic believed there was more than what he could see with his eyes.

All our memories and beliefs make up our personal bio-system we call self: body, mind and emotions. In fact, our bodies are made of frequency. The atoms and molecules have a frequency, and everything we see or hear is in effect, to an extent, of that frequency. Everything we think contributes to that frequency. In this way, we are self-made, but only so within a larger context of a life-Source that is the stuff with which we co-create, stuff we can term, with our limited words, *consciousness, thought* and *matter*.

Our very commonly accepted tools of desire and thought, and our beliefs, so overlooked and taken for granted, are the very powers we use to make a life of illness or health. As it turns out, we can give ourselves health.

As Bernie Siegel, M.D., notes in his fine article, we can open ourselves to health. Deepak Chopra, M.D., raises a point in his "Healing the Quantum Heart": "In theory, the mind can cure any disease." Let's explore a bit of that healing mind in this book. Can it be simple to recognize the wholeness of health? Does one only need believe it to be there and feel it? As a great mystic once said, "There is more knowing in the felt sense of wholeness than words can ever teach."

—S.M.

The mind is its own place, and in itself Can make a Heav'n of Hell, a Hell of Heav'n.

—"Paradise Lost," Milton

Spiritual Aspects of the Healing Arts

Bernie Siegel, M.D., with Barbara H. Siegel

IN AN INTUITIVE WAY, I believe from the time life begins one is aware of the true nature of healing, or the fact that it is not mechanical or remedy oriented. A mother's touch, kiss, or a doctor's phone call suddenly bring relief. We begin to become aware of the interplay of psyche and soma.

From the outset one must understand that all healing is scientific. The problem is science's inability to measure or document what occurs. A typical example is the so-called spontaneous remission of an incurable cancer. 3I would rather have this spontaneous event retitled "creative or self-induced healing," or "hard work miracle." The former title turns aside the health practitioner's curiosity, since it doesn't fit his scientific knowledge or his belief system. Solzhenitsyn wrote of self-induced healing in *Cancer Ward* (Farrar, Straus, Giroux, 1969):

> Kostoglotov . . . [said] . . . "we shouldn't behave like

rabbits and put our complete trust in doctors. For instance, I'm reading this book." He picked up a large, open book from the window sill. "Abriksosov and Stryukov, *Pathological Anatomy*, medical school textbook. It says here that the link between the development of tumors and the central nervous system has so far been very little studied. And this link is an amazing thing! It's written here in so many words." He found the place. "'It happens rarely, but there are cases of self-induced healing.' You see how it's worded? Not recovery through treatment, but actual healing. See?"

There was a stir throughout the ward. It was as though "self-induced healing" had fluttered out of the great open book like a rainbow-colored butterfly for everyone to see, and they all held up their foreheads and cheeks for its healing touch as it flew past.

"Self-induced." said Kostoglotov, laying aside his book. He waved his hands, fingers splayed. . . . "That means that suddenly for some unexplained reason the tumor starts off in the opposite direction! It gets smaller, resolves and finally disappears! See?"

They were all silent, gaping at the fairy tale. That a tumor, one's own tumor, the destructive tumor which had mangled one's whole life, should suddenly drain away, dry up and die by itself?

The were all silent, still holding their faces up to the butterfly. It was only the gloomy Podduyev who made his bed creak and, with a hopeless and obstinate expression on his face, croaked out, "I suppose for that you need to have . . . a clear conscience."

To understand how to fit spirituality into the healing process or to recognize its place, let me take a step back and describe present medical training.

Young men and women are accepted into medical school based upon their ability to take tests and accumulate knowledge. (Hopefully they also have an interest in people.) They are then taught about disease and its treatment. Little if any time is given to the study of their feelings and how to deal with people.

They are oriented into a failure system, meaning, we fill our time, offices and hospitals with people who don't do well, and we do more to them if their first treatment fails. We fight disease with the poor patient as the battleground. If a patient does well, we do not see him again, and if he gets well when he is not supposed to, we tell him it isn't necessary for him to return, or ignore his recovery as being mystical. Any good business would study success, but medicine ignores it. We should be knocking on survivors' doors saying, "Why didn't you die when you were supposed to?" We should be teaching the messages all survivors know. By survivors, I mean survivors of disease, concentration camps, tragic life events, or other disasters.

The students become more mechanics than healers. They are taught what to do to people who are sick and little about why people get sick. They are, therefore, given the unspoken role of lifesavers. Again, this sets them up for failure, since everyone ultimately dies. The healthcare provider, therefore, withdraws from the patient so the eventual failures will be less painful. He, therefore, does not become aware of what truly occurs when one lives with disease. He has little contact with the healing process or its absence. The disease can never become a motivator for change in this setting.

I felt very unhappy as a mechanic-lifesaver. I knew from my childhood that there was more to the healing process. I knew doctors were not always right in sentencing people to death. My mother was told not to become pregnant or she would die. A case of hyperthyroidism had her weighing ninety pounds, and an obstetrician thought a pregnancy would be life threatening.

To make a long story short, she found another obstetrician who agreed to work with her if she gained weight. After she gained thirty pounds she conceived. I was born, and the hyperthyroidism disappeared. It was hard for me to not be accepted and loved by my parents after a beginning like that. In any event, this love was a handicap for a doctor, as it didn't fit into the medical model to which I was exposed. Nowhere in medical school was any time spent discussing why one becomes a doctor. I practiced medicine for a decade with a heavy heart, trying to fit love and spirituality into my practice. I inquired into other professions for a possible career change until a cancer patient made me aware of the people for whom I was caring. As strange as this may sound, I saw diseases in the waiting room, not people. Once I began to orient my practice to people, my life and my practice changed. Patients came in and said, "Now I can talk to you." When my belief system changed it was safe for them to talk about the spiritual and mystical events related to their illnesses.

Initially, I sent letters to one hundred patients, inviting them to begin meeting in groups to deal with their lives with an holistic approach. I expected hundreds of responses and had only twelve. I realized that of the people I saw, and see, with chronic or catastrophic illness, about twenty-percent are the truly exceptional patients or survivors. This may vary in different living areas, depending on how independent and how used to participating in their own lives they are. The exceptional patient or survivor is willing to take responsibility for his problem.

FOUR QUESTIONS

TO LEARN ABOUT the kind of person I was dealing with, I began to ask four simple questions. 1) Do you want to live to be 100? (A simple question about feeling in control and looking forward to life.) 2) What does your disease mean to you? (Is it a challenge or a death sentence? 3) Why did you need the illness? (What is it providing you with? Nurturing and love, as do our sick days at work?) 4) What happened in the year or two before you became sick? (This lets the patients know how they participate in an illness by not meeting their own needs. It makes them responsible for change if they wish to accept the responsibility.)

The mechanic would treat the illness and not look at who was sick. The healer/teacher says, "Who are you? Who were you? And what brings you to this point?" We have the opportunity to lead people on new pathways to assist them all with their rebirth.

Illness or pain is a message to change. In an all inclusive way, I used the phrase, "Everyone has his cancer, either emotional or physical." From this ground we have the option to either promote change and healing, or see it as a catastrophe or death sentence. I choose the former, and I offer it to my patients.

Since the medical profession is failure-oriented, it

11

tends to say to people, "Don't ask why you became ill"; it will make you feel that it is your fault, that you are a failure." I say the illness must be seen as a message to redirect your life, and, within this transformation, healing occurs.

I know the power of this transformation and the knowledge our inner voices, intuition, or unconscious minds can provide. For years I ignored it, but I kept getting a powerful personal message to uncover something. As a mechanic, therefore, I went to the barber and had my head shaved. Of course, having a bare head didn't solve the problem.

TWO TEACHERS

TWO TEACHERS HELPED ME. (When you are ready, a teacher will appear.) One was Elisabeth Kubler-Ross who, at a workshop, interpreted a spontaneous drawing of mine. It shows a fish out of water (a spiritual symbol) and a mountain covered with snow. (A white crayon utilized to portray snow on an already white piece of paper represents a symbolic cover-up.) What this drawing did was to show me what needed to be uncovered was not my head but my love and spirituality, and then I would no longer feel like a fish out of water. Prior to meeting Elisabeth, I attended a workshop with Carl and Stephanie Simonton and was told during a guided imagery exercise I would meet an inner guide. The mechanic in me said, "This is all ridiculous." And yet, in the meditation, along came George. George is a spiritual figure who guides me. Since then I have met other guides who have been seen by mediums. I only see the guides in imagery exercises and sense them around me, but mediums have seen them standing around me at my lectures or workshops. A new world opened up where a mechanic could exist no longer with his old belief system. By bringing this new belief system into my practice, my world, and the world of my patients changed. I realized that mind and body communicate by a symbolic language, and consequently I now utilize dreams and drawings as a regular part of my therapeutic and diagnostic approach. Mind, body, and spirit are considered as one unit. Being a highly skilled mechanic is important, but true healing occurs only when psyche, soma and spirit are integrated.

When you use this new approach, patients begin to share with you the life events prior to their becoming ill. They realize the illness allows them to say no to demands they would have felt obligated to fulfill. However, when I offer people options for getting well, most prefer the mechanical, "Cut it out, I can get a babysitter" approach, instead of one of changing their lifestyle. They say exercise and meditation may change family routine, and the spouse will be angry.

> We would rather be ruined than changed.
> We would rather die in our dread
> than climb the cross of the moment and
> let our illusions die. —W.H. Auden

The illness gives me a chance to teach people about unconditional love: giving with no expectations because one chooses to give. Discipline and saying no are permitted between two people sharing this love. It is the conditional love upon which most of us are brought up that leads to illness. We never get all the "thank yous" and praise we would like. It is having something to give that restores us and provides us with a reason for living, when what we are giving is unconditional love. Physical handicap or illness

13

does not interfere with the ability to give love. Invariably the love is returned to us without our asking because people see the change and want to be closer to this new found peace.

Many of my patients who are physically quite ill, some near death, wonder why they still have so many visitors. I explain to them that their spirit is very much alive and that "terminal" is a state of mind. Their spirit and love attract others because the others see life, not death, and therefore are comfortable in their presence.

In 1926 Elida Evans, in her book entitled *A Psychological Study of Cancer* said, "Cancer is a symbol, as most illness is, of something going wrong in the patient's life, a warning to him to take another road." Those who take this new road find a new life, exceed expectations and sometimes are cured of incurable illness. The new lifestyle is the goal, not physical well-being. The latter is the traditional medical approach.

PHYSICIAN AS SPIRITUAL LEADER

THE PHYSICIAN CAN BE A SPIRITUAL LEADER and help people be reborn. These same patients are not upset with you for not healing them physically, but they actually thank you for the new life and ability to love. They feel this way because you indeed have made them eternal in the only way possible.

The secret to being eternal is love. Thornton Wilder said, "... and we ourselves shall be loved for a while and then forgotten, but the love will have been enough, even memory is not necessary for love. There is a land of the living and a land of the dead, and the bridge is love." It can be said in another way: to die, but not to perish, that is eternity. Love teaches us how not to perish.

There is eternal life through love, yet part of the reason physicians have no need to deal with this problem is that unconsciously they believe doctors don't get sick or die. (This is an unconscious reason for many to become doctors, but it is never addressed during medical training. There is a massive denial that keeps them from feeling what their patients feel and, therefore, from needing to face illness and death. For those who face these problems, the physician has little advice. When I asked God what to do when confronted with a patient with a serious illness who I could help, or God could heal, He said "Render unto the doctor what is the doctor's and unto God what is God's."

One patient, when confronted with a dismal future leading to the grave, asked her doctor (who made the prognosis), "But what can I do?" He replied, "You only have a hope and a prayer." She asked, "How do I hope and pray?" And he said, "I don't know, that's not my line of work." With my help she has learned to hope and pray. She has transcended her physical illness and her fears, and now she goes to her doctor to bring him life and love. He, incidentally, has become very busy making notes about her exceptional course.

Doctors' invulnerability is one aspect of the problem, and another is what I have labeled the "war and peace" aspect of medicine. The doctor sees God as coming in only when he feels helpless or hopeless, an unfortunate loss of the spiritual component of healing. Spirituality should not be relegated to "helpless" cases, because it provides exceptional results, and has cured the medically incurable.

Where can spirituality fit into a war on disease? How does the greatest healing power in the universe adjust to killing? Can healing occur in this environment? Listen to the language of medicine's war on illness: we kill, insult, assault, blast, and poison you and your body. All these are words with which doctors are comfortable. Tests have shown that eighty percent of all people are not comfortable killing, unless they have to kill to save the lives of loved ones. Neither are we comfortable in killing disease, since it is a part of us. There is only a small percentage of patients who are comfortable being aggressive toward something residing within.

The disease should be seen as a part of a personal growth process. We can use our white blood cells to consume the disease (nourish themselves on the disease) and we can grow psychologically because of the disease. This process then creates immune system changes that can lead us to healing and new life.

I believe diseases are a response to loss, and I have often thought of the comparison to a salamander. Salamanders, incidentally, have few cancers, but do have the ability to regenerate, and we have the opposite potential.

If a salamander has a loss, it grows a new part. If we have a loss, we grow a cancer or generate a disease. As one of my patients said, "I grew it to fill the emptiness inside of me."

If a salamander has an extensive cancer and its tail is cut off, a new tail grows, and the cancer returns to normal cells. By instructing my patients to grow, I hope to stop the growth within them, restore them to normal and open a pathway to physical, mental and spiritual health.

My therapeutic goal has more to do with peace of mind than physical healing. Why? Because that is the stuff of which miracles are made. W.C. Ellerbroek, former surgeon and now psychiatrist, feels that cancer miracles occur only when people are moribund, or practically so. That is when they give up the despair, and the healing process begins. (He has over five dozen well-documented cases at last communication.) How sad to wait until one is almost dead to resolve conflict.

I try to teach this message to my patients. Live with a sense of time limitation. Decide things based upon the value of your time. Say what needs to be said, resolve conflicts, and share openly the love you feel. What happens then?

One of my hospitalized patients told me she felt like dying. I said, "That's all right, but please share this feeling with your children and your parents. They don't know how badly you feel." I came back after the weekend to see her, and she looked wonderful. She had on make-up, a suit and her wig. I said, "What happened?" She answered, "I told my children how I felt. I told my parents how I felt, and then I felt so good I didn't want to die." She was discharged from the hospital. I have seen other patients who were expected to die resolve their conflicts and be discharged with, as one patient said, "incredible energy." That is the power of love which resides in each of us. I have watched those who have learned to live leave their bodies. It is a peaceful, pain-free process in which no time is really spent dying. It is a letting go. For this to occur two basic conditions must be met. The lifesaver/doctor must be instructed when to stop, and loved ones must give permission to the individual with the illness to fight or not. Finally, those with the illness are given permission to die when they no longer feel they are "living." Their survivors share their love and grief and the knowledge that they will be able to go on because of the shared love. This allows the life and death decision to be made by the individual, free from the "don't die" messages we often give each other. If we give "don't die" messages death becomes a failure, something that must occur in secret when the loved ones and lifesavers are not present.

This then allows the individual the choice not only of a time to die but also of people with whom the event is shared. It allows them to see their loved one take one breath and die.

Being present at such a death makes one aware that it is a transition. The spirit leaves the body, the cocoon, and moves on. Scientists will describe this as the parasympathetic nervous system slowing and stopping bodily functions, but it doesn't look scientific, it looks spiritual when you are there.

Just as Solzhenitsyn, in his book *Cancer Ward*, sees spontaneous healing as a rainbow colored butterfly, so his unconscious knows that to heal, one must deal with one's life spectrum (the rainbow), shed the cocoon, and become a new person (a butterfly) with a "clear conscience" as Podduyef says in the book.

This spontaneous change can more easily occur when we open to God's healing energy. Once a patient of mine returned to the office free of an incurable cancer and said, "I left my troubles to God." I now had a therapy to share with others.

However, if God said to you "be happy!" what would most of us do? We would ask for an exception in our case. Why? Because if God only knew our life and troubles, He wouldn't ask us to be happy; He would allow us to be victims and an exception to his rule of happiness.

CREATING A HEALING ENVIRONMENT

IF ONE CONCEIVES OF GOD as intelligent, love and light, and if one opens to this light, true healing of mind, body and spirit can occur. My fantasy is that someday our nuclear physicists will become our theologians when they discover this ultimate source of intelligent, loving energy. A new specialty of theological physics will then exist.

I have long felt the absence of God from our hospitals. Notice the absence of signs of spirituality in a hospital not run by a religious order. One of my associates, Richard Selzer, a surgeon and writer, shares my feeling eloquently in his short story "Absence of Windows." He states, "I very much fear that, having bricked up our windows, we have lost more than the breeze; we have severed a celestial connection." In this article he was discussing the removal of the windows from the operating room.

19

How do we reestablish this connection? Obviously not by bringing windows back, but by creating a healing, spiritual environment. I personally use music as a way of reestablishing this connection. Since biblical times this quality of music has been known. It creates a mental state conducive to healing, as well as a greater awareness of the true nature of healing and our common source.

It is my belief that music creates a healing rhythm within the body, a harmony of all parts. I believe dreams and drawings reveal the symbolism of this rhythm. Healthy organs have their natural vibration based upon their molecular structure.

Disease changes this rhythm; disharmony occurs, and it registers in the mind. To convert this to mental awareness, symbols are used. If we pay attention to these symbolic messages we can diagnose disease at an earlier stage and, hopefully, learn to send healing messages or symbols back to the body. Historically, Carl Jung diagnosed physical illness based upon patients' dreams. And I have been able to do so with dreams or drawings. Frequently the patients are already aware of the dream contents and meaning, and are simply sharing it with me. My patients' dreams and drawings reveal our common or collective unconscious, our common origin, our shared beginning with all men, and so the source of healing is of the same origin for us all.

What are the changes which create this environment conducive to healing?: The introduction of laughter, music, love, forgiveness and acceptance—all coming after a release of resentment, conflict and despair. Every cell in the body is then involved in the healing process. When we laugh every cell laughs. When we love, our immune system feels the most vibrant, live message it can receive, and it fights for our life. I say choose this course not in an attempt to try to live forever, but because of the beauty it brings to your life. It is God's work. If you choose to love you are a success. You will have days when you will disappoint yourself for not loving enough, but forgive and go on. It is the pilgrimage which is important and what we encounter along the way; not the necessity of reaching "sainthood," but striving toward it. Emmett Fox has said,

> There is no difficulty that enough love will not conquer; no disease that enough love will not heal; no door that enough love will not open; no gulf that enough love will not bridge; no wall that enough love will not throw down; no sin that enough love will not redeem. . . .
>
> It makes no difference how deeply seated may be the trouble; how hopeless the outlook; how muddled the tangle; how great the mistake. A sufficient realization of love will dissolve it all. If only you could love enough you would be the happiest and most powerful being in the world.

To me the last sentence is the key. Some of us may feel like failures if we don't accomplish everything he suggests, but it is the exceptional person who chooses to attempt it and knows how hard it is. Yet it is this difficulty that allows us through shared pain to help each other. The person who chooses to be the family failure or life's victim is no help to others. He is always dying. Lovers are always living and feeling. Rilke has said, "Do not believe that he who seeks to comfort you lives untroubled among the simple and quiet words that sometimes do you good. His life has much difficulty and sadness and remains far behind yours. Were it otherwise he would never have been able to find those words."

To choose love is to bring into effect the spiritual healing force and source of life. I choose to live by Teilhard de Chardin's words. "Someday, after we have mastered the winds, the waves, the tides, and gravity, we shall harness for God the energies of love. Then, for the second time in the history of the world man will have discovered fire."

One could go on quoting the great men of history referring to the power of love and not convince anyone. I say to all of you, believe and see the change that occurs in your lives, or spend a lifetime being convinced and never seeing.

Science teaches us to see in order to believe, and the spirit says believe and you will see. I know the latter to be true.

LIFE AFTER LIFE

IN MY EARLY YEARS of practice, patients did not share either their healing or out of body and life after life experiences, and I wondered if any of this was true. When I changed my patients changed. Of course it was my change. Now they were free to share with a believer. A blind patient seeing as he watched his own resuscitation—an amputee being whole again and describing the beauty of where we are all going. Many of my patients have shared these incredibly moving and beautiful experiences that again remove fear and fill their lives with love. Their bodies being God's gifts, they use them to the fullest before choosing to move on.

One patient of mine, a physician, was naturally very scientific and found it all hard to believe. When I asked him one day in the hospital, when he was quite ill, if he were ready to die, he said, "Considering the alternative, no." Three months after his death, a student came to interview me and gave me a card containing a message. She said she had been at a healing circle and told everyone she was going to interview me the following day. The medium present asked if there were a message for Dr. Siegel, and she wrote out the message she received on the card. The card said, "To Bernie from Frank, love and peace. If I had known it were this easy I'd have bought the package a long time ago, I wouldn't have resisted so much." The language on the card was Frank's way of referring to my teachings. He had never, "bought the package."

To be handed this note helped me to believe. I only ask others to be open to this in their own lives and to see what occurs. Let this intuitive guiding force lead you on the correct path. I instruct my students that when they are on this path they will know; elevator doors will open without pushing the button, and people will appear whom you plan to call.

One stops judging what I call "spiritual flat tires," which are those events that delay you in order for you to meet someone you wouldn't have met if you had not had the "flat tire" event. I ask you to believe and see what occurs in your life. Live with a sense of time limitation, and, because of it, feel comfortable to say no—without guilt.

23

Love, be selfless, childlike, and see the love returned to you.

CONCLUSION

I CAN SAY that my initial attempt to help twelve of my patients (disciples), in our first "exceptional cancer patient" group, has led me to receive love from several continents. I have had the opportunity to love and heal so many more, including medical students and physicians, who are opening to this new light all because I wanted to give something to the world.

I would like to continue to share with all of you, but space obviously limits the number of anecdotes and metaphors that can be included. Let me close with two quotes by Carl Jung, whose work I consider one of my greatest resources. "Your picture of God or your idea of immortality is atrophied, consequently your psychic metabolism is out of gear." and, "Every problem therefore, brings the possibility of a widening of consciousness, but also the necessity of saying goodbye to childlike unconsciousness and trust in nature."

It is time for medicine to get its psychic metabolism in gear and cast aside the guilt caused by leaving the garden of eden (trust in nature). We must become a success oriented healing discipline using the patient's illness as the "ticket of admission." Then, not mechanics, but healers and teachers will redirect their lives on a healing pathway. You might ask me why I am still a surgeon. I still see my mechanical skills as a way of buying time for the healing process to happen. I know I can operate on patients and see them have less pain and fewer complications when we are a healing team, utilizing faith in ourselves, our treatment and our spiritual faith. Despite all that has been said up to this point, as a surgeon my feet remain on the ground. Patients do have complications and do die, but in the process I still have something to offer them. The mechanic would be at a loss and would probably desert them.

In closing, let me share a few words from a traditional Indian saying that sums up my message. "When you were born, you cried and the whole world rejoiced. Live such a life, that when you die the whole world cries and you rejoice." To accomplish this requires only a short time. As long as one is alive it can be accomplished; change can occur. Richard Bach, the author of *Jonathan Livingston Seagull* has said, "Here is a test to find if your mission on earth is finished. If you're alive it isn't." Many children who die give the gift of love to their parents and it lasts them a lifetime. Others choose a lifetime of hate because of a similar loss. I can only ask, as the Bible does, for you to choose life.

> If I am not for myself, who will be?
> If I am only for myself, what am I?
> If not now, when?   —Martin Buber Δ

Although our society is trying its best to deny it, we are whole people with spiritual as well as physical and mental natures.

—George Hogben, M.D.

Can You Decide When to Get Sick—And When Not to?

Blair Justice, Ph.D.

IF YOU ARE IN THE BIG MIDDLE of an all-important project—requiring your very best under the pressure of too little time—and you tell yourself you simply cannot let yourself get sick from the stress, will your body listen and allow you to postpone illness?

Some people believe that by talking to their bodies, they can keep from getting sick until a more convenient time. Others notice that they often work well and feel good while under stress, but they invariably become ill afterward. Does this kind of experience also support the idea that illness can be deferred—or are there people who actually need to stay under stress to stay well?

27

The answer to each of these questions seems to be yes, if the findings now coming out of a wide range of stress research hold up. Not only is there reason to believe that people can—and do—defer stress-related illness, but also there is growing evidence to suggest that stress can give a boost to the body as well as inflict damage.

What stress does, good or bad, to our health is becoming clearer as researchers learn more about how the brain and its neurotransmitters affect the body's glands, hormones, cardiovascular system and immune cells. Although scientists on all levels of biomedical research, from the molecular to the behavioral, have failed to arrive at a common definition for stress, most would agree with Dr. John Mason, Yale neuroendocrinologist, that the term "strikes some deep, responsive chord within us" and is assured of survival "in spite of all the confusion it creates" in science.

In other words, while people may use the word *stress* differently—some referring to the demands and pressure in our lives and others to how it makes us feel—most are convinced it can have profound effects on our health. The excitement today comes from the burgeoning evidence on what happens in the brain and body that helps explain some of the intriguing paradoxes of stress. For example:

—Changes do occur in the body when people talk to their hurting parts and stabilize their autonomic or "involuntary" nervous system—the system largely responsible for the stress response and the one that regulates many of our internal organs.

—High levels of catecholamines in the brain—

neurotransmitters like epinephrine (adrenaline) that have a stimulating effect—can keep people who are intensely focused on what they are doing from noticing they are injured or getting sick.

—People who are fiercely determined to stay healthy or alive until a specified time seem to mobilize self-repair systems, only dimly understood, that enable them to do what they vowed.

—Some people who work long hours and never take a vacation have such a passion for what they are doing, and such control over it, that they may seldom feel any stress or get sick.

—Those who become ill after an intense period of stress, which may have even been stimulating or exciting, often experience a steady elevation of stress hormones that can depress their immune system.

—The immune system is also affected by the body's own opioids or "opiates"—endorphins and enkephalins—and whether they lower immunity or raise it may depend on how much control a person perceives over stress and its effects.

—A sense of control—particularly the ability to control how we look at demanding or troubling situations as well as react to them—seems a central key to whether the effects of stress on the body are good or bad.

Those who stave off their symptoms by talking to their bodies enhance this sense of control when they see the effects they can have on their own physiology. "A few years ago they would have been considered a little crazy," noted Dr. Anees Sheikh at a conference in St. Louis sponsored by the American Imagery Institute and the Medical College of Wisconsin. Dr. Sheikh is a professor of psychology and chairman of the department at Marquette University.

Findings from his laboratory as well as research at Stanford University, the Yale Behavioral Medicine Clinic and elsewhere have shown that the perceptions people make, the pictures they put in their heads and the words they say to themselves all have physiological consequences. In fact, the cognitions and images themselves seem to constitute electrochemical events in the brain on the molecular level.

What goes on at this level is important because biomedical scientists use a molecular theory of disease to explain the mechanisms and processes by which people get sick. When someone, for instance, develops ulcers from excessive secretion of hydrochloric acid, one of the mechanisms producing this result involves stomach cells— parietal cells—that have receptors—called H2 receptors— for histamine molecules. Histamine is one of many messenger molecules in the body that carry on communication among cells. A messenger communicates by acting like a key that fits the configuration of the molecules on the surface or membrane of a receiving cell. The histamine molecules fit the particular shape of the receptor "locks" of parietal cells and turn on a series of biochemical events that results in hydrochloric acid secretion. The success of the widely used drug cimetidine in treating ulcers comes from making its molecular configuration closely resemble the structure of histamine so that the drug will occupy the parietal "locks" and keep the offending messenger from having any receptors to key into.

When our hypothalamus triggers the stress response and activates neurotransmitters, hormones and other messenger molecules in the brain and body, these substances in turn act on the receptors of the heart, blood vessels, muscles and—as recently established—immune cells, which protect us from bacteria and viruses. When too many "keys" are finding their way into too many "locks," the heart races, blood presssure increases, muscles tighten, and immunity can be suppressed if the stress continues. If we keep evoking our stress response and ignore it, or do nothing about it, the consequence may be that we get sick or find ourselves in pain.

But how does talking to the body help—and what do people actually say to hurting parts?

"You can ask the pain to leave now," said Dr. Sheikh. "You can tell it to come back in two hours, or two days, when you can listen to it and see what it is telling you."

A nurse at the imagery conference who said she uses this technique to defer symptoms commented: "I get headaches under stress. I acknowledge the pain and say, 'Please leave, I'm busy now. I'll tend to you later.' When I do this three times, it goes away."

A psychologist remarked: "I say to my stomach: 'Hi, stomach. What's the matter? Let's talk.' " The hypothalamus, which takes orders from the thoughts, words and images we put in higher centers of the brain, can turn on a relaxation response in the body as well as a stress reaction. This may be one way that soothing talk to the body helps.

At Yale, Dr. Gary Schwartz has been talking up the benefits of self-attention ever since he became convinced that disregulation of the autonomic nervous system often occurs from failure to keep mind and body "connected." When we ignore our stress or do nothing about it, the feedback loops that normally keep our biochemical and neural processes in balance become disconnected. Just giving some conscious attention to the body is often enough to restore connection and stabilize the system, according to Dr. Schwartz, who is director of the Yale Behavioral Medicine Clinic.

In a master series lecture for the American Psychological Association, Dr. Schwartz told of a 3-year-old boy treated at the clinic for serious migraine headaches. Using temperature biofeedback, the child became adept at warming his hands and decreased his daytime headaches by more than eighty percent. Research has shown that if blood vessels in the hands can be kept dilated, those in the head that often constrict at the start of migraines will also remain open. On his own, the little boy started commanding his hands to get warm by saying out loud: "Hands—you're hot!" In one to two minutes his hands would warm by ten to fifteen degrees.

Talking to the body to stave off symptoms or reduce effects of the stress response works best after a person has taken some form of relaxation or biofeedback training. But to prove his point about how giving attention to the body will help regulate the autonomic nervous system and counteract stress effects, Dr. Schwartz invited psychologists at his lecture to close their eyes for a minute and pay attention to their breathing. Most agreed that their breathing became slower, deeper and more regular. The very process of noticing one's breathing, Dr. Schwartz said, is often enough to connect mind and body and stabilize the autonomic nervous system.

People who pay attention to their bodies and have high personal consciousness tend to show greater resistance to stress and illness than do those who seldom monitor themselves. In a study at State University of New York at Albany, Dr. Jerry Suls and Barbara Fletcher found that stressful life events predicted illness in persons low in self-attention but not in those who scored high on this quality.

When our stress response is constantly being triggered, the autonomic nervous system keeps the body aroused with stimulation from stress hormones and other chemicals. For some people, the arousal—primarily from epinephrine and norepinephrine—can be such a heady experience they may not even notice they are injured or have tissue damage. Shirley MacLaine, in one of her books, tells of performing a ballet on point with a broken ankle. Dr. Errol Korn, a gastroenterologist and specialist in pain management on the clinical faculty at the University of California, San Diego, recalled at the imagery conference that in recent Olympic competition, a Japanese gymnast broke his tibia doing a flip twist dismount, then went on to perform his next routine so well that he won a silver medal.

Release of natural opiates in the body, which often occurs in the brain after stress chemicals peak, do not seem to explain failure to notice injury as much as the intense focus on the challenge of performance and the stimulating effects of catecholamines.

People who get sick after concentrated perioods of pressure at work may also raise their stress hormones to levels that, for a time, keep "the juices flowing" freely and performance at an optimum. But sooner or later, limits that each individual has are likely to be reached, and the person leaves the "resistance" stage of the stress response and enters exhaustion. Interestingly, the peaking—and then declining—of stress hormones and the loss of resistance may not occur until the pressure period is over. Dr Marianne Frankenhaueser, pioneer psychobiologist at the University of Stockholm and Karolinska Institute in Sweden, studied aftereffects of stress in a group of female employees who put in seventy-three hours of extra work over two months, with most of the overtime occurring in a two-week period. Their maximum work load was in the middle of the overtime period but their peak epinephrine (adrenaline) output was at the end. Even at home at nights, the women had pronounced stress hormone levels.

Peak catecholamine levels, after extended stress, may be followed by the onset of symptoms of respiratory disorders and infectious diseases. Dr. William Gruchow at the University of Waterloo in Ontario found that symptoms tended to occur three days after the elevated levels. Because high levels of stress hormones can suppress the immune system, increased susceptibility to colds, coughs and flu may be the price paid later for an all-out push at work.

One of the intriguing effects of strong surges of norepinephrine in the brain seems to be that people remember in great detail their stressful episode or experience. Areas of the brain involved in memory—primarily the hippocampus and amygdala—may become so "sensitized" or "potentiated" that any small cue reminds a person of what had earlier been experienced and evokes stress symptoms.

But whether we get sick after stress also depends on how much the body needs a break from deadlines, appointments and social obligations for awhile. Part of each individual's threshold for stress has to do with his or her "organ reserve"—capacity to function properly—which can be exceeded by trying to do too much, too long, too fast.

Another influence on the aftereffects of stress is our exposure to germs. Although it is true that lowered immunity may result in illness because bacteria or viruses already in the body become activated, people may nevertheless raise their risks by staying cooped up in offices or apartments, where others are more likely to pass on germs. Making a point to spend time outdoors after stress may reduce exposure, says Dr. Wolfgang Vogel, professor of pharmacology and psychiatry at Jefferson Medical College in Philadelphia.

The best news, though, is that sickness after stress is avoidable for many people. In a study of more than one-hundred middle-managers and executives of Illinois Bell Telephone, Dr. Suzanne Kobasa and her colleagues at the University of Chicago found that—even in the midst of

AT&T divestiture and its attendant stresses—about half the group stayed free of illness. They were distinguished by three factors: (1) an ability to look at change as a challenge and not a threat; (2) an ability to be optimistic and to deal with problems with a sense of control, and (3) a strength and sense of involvement that comes from commitment to work, family and friends. Such stress resistance—termed "personality hardiness"—can be taught to people, the researchers determined, and in follow-up studies of hundreds of executives, they found that it provides more protection against illness than even physical exercise, social support or a strong constitution.

The control people experience in the face of stress seems to be greatly enhanced once they learn that they can markedly influence what happens in their bodies by how they view problems. Research has shown that "awfulizing"—viewing demands and difficulties as horrible and terrible—only increases the intensity of stress experienced and the risk of damage suffered. Recent studies by Dr. Vogel support both experimental and clinical evidence that the effect of stress on the immune system—on natural killer cells that protect against cancer as well as T and B cells that fight infectious disease—is strongly infleunced by a person's sense of control. The beauty to acquiring this kind of control—which is more cognitive than behavioral—is that it does not depend on doing away with the external problem; it comes from controlling what the problem does to us. By reducing the impact or intensity of our stress, we are then better able to deal with the external problem.

Although the research is in its infancy, a sense of control may also help explain the exciting new findings of Dr. Nicholas Plotnikoff, another professor of pharmacology, who has come up with a "yin-yang hypothesis" on immune defenses. He has found that whether the endorphins and enkephalins released during stress are "up regulators"—which enhance our immune system—or "down regulators"—which impair it—depends on which of four receptors (delta, epsilon, mu or kappa) they bind to on T cells. Their preference may be at least partly determined by how well we cope, which usually amounts to how much control we perceive. Dr. Plotnikoff is on the faculty at the University of Illinois at Chicago.

Another way to enhance control over the stress response and its effects is to learn relaxation exercises and imagery techniques. Dr. Korn, who teaches both, notes that for the past twelve years—since he himself began practicing the techniques—he has not had even a cold although his scores on stress scales are extremely high (more than 1,000 on the Holmes-Rahe life events scale, which he takes twice annually). "It's not the stressors that are important but how you react to them and what you do about them," he told the conference in St. Louis.

Dr. Korn recently studied "hyper-performers" in business and public life—people like Lee Iacocca, Margaret Thatcher, Ed Koch, Bob Hope, Michael DeBakey—and concluded that a passion for work can be healthy. As observed a long time ago by Dr. Hans Selye, the most widely quoted stress researacher of all, some people are "racehorses" and need high stimulation to stay well. Others are "turtles" and require less stress.

Most of us are probably in between. But understanding why we get sick when we do may move us a step closer to that charmed circle of both racehorses and turtles who not only defer illness from stress but prevent it as well. Δ

Thoughts can heal the body because thoughts created its need to be healed.

—Anon

Thoughts and the Roots of Health

Scott Miners

THOUGHTS MANIFEST AS LIFE. Your thoughts and my thoughts. Remember the well-known statement, "In the beginning was the word?" Change it. It should read, "In the beginning was the thought." The radical findings of many pioneering researchers in the fields of neuroscience, medicine and what has been termed "molecular psychology" indicate that every thought we think in some way affects our bodies—for its health and joy or lack of it. Every thought. Something in my conscience bothers me as I read their data. They have what seems to be incontrovertible evidence that we provide ourselves with our own health—or separate ourselves from it—by what we think.

We can give ourselves health or take it away by what we think. What kind of responsibility is this? "You mean I cannot blame my parents or some outer determinant any more for any ill-health I may perceive in my body? I cannot blame, if not my heredity, a God who sits on a celestial throne and gives health to one but not another? I am a thinking and co-creating force in my world?" What is the evidence supportive of what seems to be such a departure from the messages in our culture that something outside of us determines our health or our lack of it? And, were those messages true in the first place? Have we always played a role in co-determining our own health? What is the evidence?

Let's look at some basic facts. Neuroscientist Alexis Traynor-Kaplan, from the University of California at San Diego Medical School, works with intracellular signal transduction—the examination of the way information is transferred (in our case, in a human body) from the surface of a cell to the inside of a cell.[1] This is analogous to someone making a phone call from one office to another inside a large skyscraper. Traynor-Kaplan notes that part of the way the mind communicates with (makes phone calls to) the body and the body to itself is by way of hormones and neurotransmitters. The hormones travel through the bloodstream to cells throughout the body. The cells have receivers—called receptors—by way of which they can receive "calls," or hormones. Remember that word: *receptors*.

Neurotransmitters are slightly different. They are released from nerve endings. But, as with hormones, cells throughout the body, including the brain, have receptors for these neurotransmitters, which transmit "information."[2] Imagine, if the cell were about the size of your tongue, that a taste "bud" on your tongue would represent a cell receptor. Each area of the tongue is sensitive, or receptive to specialized chemicals in foods, thus one area of the tongue is sensitive to sour and another to sweet. The same specialization occurs in our cells. When certain hormones or neurotransmitters lock into a specialized receptor of a cell, changes can be triggered within the cell—just as a phone call from one secretary in one office can trigger change in the "receiver" of the call in another office.

Traynor-Kaplan explains that the body is a system of feedback loops connected with the brain/mind. The brain is one area where neurotransmitters and hormones are released (from such glands as the pituitary and the pineal). The brain can also send messages to organs to release hormones, as well as to glands throughout the body, such as the thyroid and the adrenals. Thought affects this activity in the brain; therefore, it can also affect the whole body through the self-regulating system of neurotransmitters and hormones. The word self-regulating is important to remember, for it is descriptive not only of the body, but also of our self-generated thoughts.

THOUGHTS AFFECT THE ACTIVITY of the brain and body in many ways. Not the least of these is the way in which a thought held in the brain can affect our emotional state. For example, let us monitor that phone call from one secretary in her office to a colleague in another office. Let's imagine that the caller, we'll call her Sara, who was not feeling very chipper in the moment, said rather flatly to the other, a close friend who we'll name Beth, "Beth, your boss is planning to let you go today." Many feelings may flood into Beth's emotions. She may have thoughts of anxiety about paying her bills, about self-esteem or even a sad memory of a previous time when she was out of work. Let's view that memory. The memory, by focusing thought on it, can trigger hormones to be released from the pituitary and other glands. Her previous unemployment was a frightening experience for Beth, so she triggered the well known adrenal release and actually recreated the physical state of fear she experienced during her first unemployment adventure. Her body went through an actual biological reaction to a thought.

As it so happens, the entire thought/emotion, or mind/brain/body event that occurred for Beth was an illusion created by her thoughts in more ways than one. Sara only meant that Beth's boss was "letting her go" early so the two of them could see a play that evening. Beth, in her busyness, had forgotten their plans momentarily, and she had reacted to the statement with several anxious thoughts and emotional states. Interestingly, this adrenal response and all emotions took place within less than fifteen seconds. Such is the power of thought to transform the biological functions, the hormonal and neuro-signalling and cellular receiving of the body. What happened to the atoms and molecules and cells in Beth's body? What happens to mine or yours every morning when we drive to work? Can we monitor our thoughts masterfully enough to be fully immune to the "slings and arrows" of our adventure in life?

Let's first look at a small portion of what happened in Beth's body. When she interpreted the communication that she was in immediate danger of losing her job, she felt stressful emotions. Everyone has different ways of coping with stress. Beth, though she has many coping skills, reacted to the stress by engaging the fight or flight response. She perceived a threat, and her pituitary gland was sent a signal (intercellular signal), by the brain, from the thought of "threat" (the thought was her inner phone call), to emit adrenocorticotrophic hormone, which stimulates the adrenal gland to emit corticosteroid hormones and epinephrine. These in turn sent more messages, which caused the pulse to increase, the muscles to tense and blood pressure to rise.

It is highly appropriate and simple to ask here, "What happens to my body/brain/mind system as I perform any number of activities in my life?" Whether I am self-employed, live in the country, am wealthy, interact with children, adults or act in any number of the millions of preferred realities human beings can have, what happens when I think, and how do my thoughts affect my health? Also, how large is the sphere of influence of my health? As physicist Sir Arthur Eddington noted, "when the electron vibrates, the universe shakes"; accordingly, when I am healthy, my biofield reverberates and affects others.

In the example of the stress experienced by Beth, the same effect takes place in other organs of the body as with the adrenal glands. Any memory you have can reenact or recreate the same biological state of the original occurence of the event that caused the memory in your body. As Traynor-Kaplan notes, you can recall the thought, or memory of childhood play and reenact or recreate some of the hormonal states in your body that existed at the time of childhood. This has the effect of rejuvenation in the body. Every series of thoughts can have emotions that occur with them, and those emotions then will signal a hormonal state with a specific set of biochemical consequences. The biochemical response of hormones and neurotransmitters as well as the cellular receptor reaction will be related to the series of thoughts regardless of whether they are from the present or from a memory. The response will vary with the vividness of the experience. Traynor-Kaplan believes that our bodies are able to rejuvenate themselves for a much longer time than what is currently considered the norm for a lifespan. It all depends upon how we feel, or the thoughts we have that transmit through the body.

It is clear that thoughts and their associated emotional states affect your body and therefore your life span. There is a great deal of literature on this subject, and I suggest you read at least the three books mentioned in reference two at the end of this article. What concerns me is the question "Why do I continue to have thoughts that seemingly do not serve the continual rejuvenation of the body? Even if I do not believe in rejuvenation, even if the neuro- and molecular sciences ascertain this or not, why would I ever think thoughts or series of them continuously, in patterns woven throughout my life span, that do not seem to serve my health? That is what bothers me as I read all of this truly awesome data—the facts about the effect of thoughts and emotional states on the equally remarkable human body at all times. At all times.

My conscience bothers me because I have begun to see that I determine, and have determined a huge portion (and, as metaphysicians of old and new ages argue all) of how my life is lived. Certainly my body runs itself by its autonomic, or self-regulating systems fascinatingly well.

But what about my self-regulation? What about my thoughts? I feel a bit in conflict and confusion knowing that I pick my thoughts, and yet I don't feel that I monitor them well enough to be a master of them. I question, "I chose my state of health? How can that be?" Let's take but a momentary diversion and look at that word *health*.

Health means "wholeness." The original and root meaning of the word is "wholeness." Logic tells me that I must therefore, in order to have health, or wholeness in my life, be aware of everything that I think. If my thoughts affect the very biological molecules of the body I inhabit in my self-expression, then it would serve me to think only thoughts that affirm the continual evolution or regeneration of those molecules—unless of course I am bored with this life and body and wish to "die," which I don't. At least not now. But wholeness also implies everything else I have ever thought. That is, all my memories and my past have led me to what I am now.[3] I am psychologically and emotionally what I have chosen to be according to my thoughts. Wholeness also implies the environment in which I (and you) live, psychologically, physically and even metaphysically—the beings we are beyond what we can see or touch.

For now, however, I want to focus only on those thoughts and emotions which have played a major role in my growth—or lack of it—for they also constrict or expand my potential. This brings us to the question of thought monitoring and the acknowledgement of the incredibly powerful and most underestimated tool we all freely have—our ability to focus upon, or choose the thoughts we think. This ability is simple and profound.

45

Using focus and choice is the way we literally co-create the world we live in and how we live in it.

For example, what can you do or say without first thinking about it? Nothing. Not one thing. Contemplate this and you will see that thought is therefore supreme, which means the thinker of the thought is also supreme. Also, as a wise friend of mine says, and this is important, our beliefs are the doorways through which everything we want in life must pass. Though as thinkers we are supreme, we direct our thoughts through our beliefs, which themselves derive from thought.

Have you ever noticed how beliefs affect health? The placebo effect is widely known. It proves in study after controlled study that what one believes becomes a reality in one's life. There are thousands of cases reported in medical literature of the placebo effect. This usually occurs in a study like the following example. A number of patients are told they are being given a new drug that has great promise for curing their particular disease. In fact, some of the patients are given the new and promising drug, and they are helped to varying degrees. Some of the patients are given a placebo, a pill that is actually made of some other substance, such as sugar, and these patients have the same rate of recovery as those who received the "real" drug. A control group is given neither drug nor placebo and the disease usually maintains its course. This "placebo effect" demonstrates clearly the power of belief.

In yet another example, a true case, a cancer patient was told a new and exciting drug had just become available that would cure him. He took the treatment and astonished his physician by being ready to leave the hospital a few days later. Weeks passed and the man went back to work and resumed a normal, healthy life, with no sign of cancer in his body. He was cured! Another month passed and his physician was notified that a mistake had been made. The drug was actually missing some vital components, and it would not have had any affect of treatment on cancerous cells at all. The physician, in his integrity, told his patient. The man's cancer returned within days and he returned to the hospital. His physician, concerned about the radical turnabout and the obvious effect of the man's beliefs, decided to tell him that the drug had been revised and was now able to help him; however, the physician gave him the same drug. The man took the "new" drug and again left the hospital when tests showed his cancerous condition was healed.

CORE BELIEFS

THERE ARE A COUNTLESS NUMBER OF BELIEFS in the world. International and national beliefs, cultural beliefs, professional beliefs, religious beliefs, familial beliefs and individual beliefs—they are usually overlapping, and they are all to be honored. They are the chosen preference of each individual, and they are the preferred realities you and I have in our lives. They are what we guage our lives by.

The placebo effect demonstrates the power and supremacy of one's own thoughts and beliefs in one's life. Of the many core beliefs we all have, one example can be seen in two pervasive beliefs about money—abundance—operating in our world. One is, "I must work hard to succeed and earn my income." Another and contrasting belief is, "I can do what I love and brings joy to me, and the money and success will surely follow." The first belief has a certain effect on my overall health; so does the second. The first may have levels of stress that are greater than the second. The first belief assumes it is hard to live. The second assumes that one is a creative being here to celebrate one's creativity, and the world is abundant and supportive. Like the lilies of the field, we will be supported. It assumes that one may imagine the unimaginable, focus on and expect fulfillment of one's desires, seek and find whatever one wishes.

What beliefs do you have? Now is a good time to make a commitment to yourself that you will set aside some time for self-examination if you have not already done so. Schedule some time on your calendar for yourself and call it "Relaxation time so that I can examine what my beliefs are." Say also, "My beliefs are powerful, and all my thoughts about my life must filter through them. There are many times in the day when I can schedule some free time for myself. I can even do this belief examination when waking in the morning, before jumping out of bed."

Will power plays a significant role in belief. Just as a wise parent would not break the will of the child, it seems to be a law of the universe that no one can break your own will. I realized after many years that no one can give me anything I don't want. If, for example, I have a belief that I need to give up or sacrifice in order to be a "good" person and merit honor from some undefined life Source, then I will sacrifice, and no one, not even that life Source, will break my will. No one could give me abundance against my belief. My beliefs fuel my will. Thus only when I allow myself the belief that "I am what I wanted," and that "I deserve love and abundance, just as does everyone else in the world," do I receive that in my life. Beliefs are that simple and powerful because through them we rule our own world. So what does this have to do with the health of the body?

The central question, since we are examining health, or wholeness, and especially the health of the bodies we all inhabit, is "What beliefs do we have about our bodies?" From there we can go on to examine all our beliefs. So, let's start at the beginning core belief about the body and its origin.

Perhaps our first response is to see images of our mothers and fathers. But I am talking about where their bodies came from and their own parents and on down the line—the Source—because that is one of the most pervasive questions. No scientist can create an acorn from which an oak tree grows, nor a body with life in it; yet, one of the most important core beliefs in life is about the life of our bodies. As was said, beliefs are the doorways through which all we want in life must pass, including our health, yet there are many conflicting beliefs about the life of the physical body.

For example, take beliefs of ultimate value. As a sort of sideline I studied world religions for many years. I was editor of a journal of comparative religion, philosophy and science, and among others I published articles from many renowned religious scholars from all over the globe. I learned about numerous central beliefs in religions that predominate for most cultures worldwide. Some of these beliefs are about the physical body and are derogatory, some few exalting, but almost without exception they view the body as being lesser than something else "out there"; something "out there" is equated to be a divine Source and creator of the life that is and animates the body. In other words, the belief is that the physical body is a lowered, or "lesser than" expression of life. Can you imagine the ripple effect of such a belief through the corridors of time, ancestry and culturally accepted conditions or rules of life?

I question that belief. What is the body lowered from, or lesser than or separate from, and how could it be "lower" if the Source of life is also the material of all the life it created?

Imagine, for those people who believe that they are "lowered," how many thoughts during the day come from this belief, thoughts like those we have seen in the example of Beth, every one of which affects the body for better or worse. How about "The physical body is separate from spirit"; "I am not good enough?" Does that one sound familiar? "My face isn't quite right"; "My legs are too short"; "I'm too heavy"; "I'm too thin" "I don't do enough for other people or love them enough—my religious authority told me so"; "I'm not worthy." Of course, I'm not worthy of life because the Source of that very life is separate from me, according to my belief, and I need to get back to it in order to be worthy, and in order to get back I have to do certain things, be good, be loving, and if I am good enough and loving enough I will be allowed back into the kingdom (of wholeness) and all will be well—but one thing is sure, I can't get there in a body.

Or can I?

I believe life has become overcomplicated. Thousands of rules have been made about how to be whole and yet, I will argue, we already are what we are told the rules will help us become—we are already whole. We're made that way. We've just forgotten.

In Hinduism there is a terse and profound story that, as spiritual beings, we assess this life and decide to be born into it, in a body, knowing exactly what it is we want to do—all we need is a body to do the active part in the physical world, which is just as "spiritual" as any world that is without physical matter. We are born. Then comes the quandry. We find ourselves as babes, not knowing. There is a veil, a forgetting. We grow up with many beliefs and rules. We now have the body, but we have forgotten our heritage and what it is we came here to do. We have forgotten our "spirituality," our oneness with spirit/Source. We forgot that life is the gift and that we are here to embrace that gift with joy; that we are spiritual beings in human bodies for the adventure of life. How does one remember? How do we go beyond limiting beliefs into the total health that is our right?

THE FIRST STEP IS TO ACKNOWLEDGE that the life which courses through our veins is sacred. Each day is. There is more knowledge in the felt experience of our being equated with the life Source than words or years of great learning can ever teach. Along with scheduling in time for self on a calendar each day for examining beliefs, we can also recognize our wholeness. Wholeness is also called God, or the Source, or the Spirit or Soul. Everything in life then becomes an effect of that feeling. Everything then becomes an effect of a core belief that we are already what perhaps we used to think was outside us to be attained. That is very empowering, and it makes life here something desired, which of course we all must have desired, else we wouldn't be here. Also, as we have seen from discussion about the power of our thoughts and beliefs, our power is not slight at all because we are in physical bodies. It exists as a potent, creative force.

Knowing that you are already whole opens up many probable realities for you in your life. Knowing that your thoughts and beliefs have profound effects on your physical health, which is your barometer for your thoughts and beliefs, is profoundly empowering. It says that you know you are in charge. This can also be frightening for some, for it places responsibility for self in one's own hands. There is all of a sudden perhaps no one to blame, no one to rely upon. But the greatest of security is knowing that the self you are is no different than that of the wholeness of the life within you. You always have that, else how would you be alive?

Enough research has been done to demonstrate the power of love in one's life and about how it affects the immune system. Now it is time to live it. A wise old friend of mine once said that love is not an emotion, it is a realization—of unity. Once you recognize that you are what perhaps before you thought was outside you only, the source within, and you recognize your heritage and that of all others, you become aware of a profound feeling of love. Schedule time for yourself for contemplation of this. All the teachings have taught about self love and how it is needed before you can love others, and how it heals all. It is time to live it.

WHERE DO YOU GO NEXT after you realize that every thought and belief you have affects your health from moment to moment? What do you do when you become aware that you can decide when to be sick and when not? As noted above, each thought you think affects the molecules of the body; each thought also affects our emotions and therefore those around us—our mates, families, friends, society and the world. Our beliefs have an equally profound effect on our health. Remember Beth and her passing belief that she had lost her job? Recall too the belief of the cancer patient in the wonder drug and then his disillusionment when he believed the drug not so wonderful—and his radical turnabout when his belief changed. Think of the placebo effect. Beliefs are powerful. Remember to schedule some time to examine your beliefs, especially your core beliefs.

I like to use the following exercise, knowing that my thoughts are powerful enough to electromagnetically and chemically affect my body—and my whole future. I like to contemplate what it is about myself I like. Believing what I say about myself is also important in this regard, as it is very difficult to truly fool myself—I know too much about me, and my conscience won't let me get away with anything. Basically this is an exercise in focusing my thoughts on what I believe I am that brings me joy. This empowers my feeling of self-love and my immune system, and since I began doing this I have enjoyed vibrant health. So have many others who I know from my counseling work and from those reports from my colleagues. I have also since enjoyed fulfilling relationships where I feel nurtured and nurturing. I have gained the self-esteem and self-respect to take myself immediately from a place where I do not feel nurtured, just as a mother would take her newborn from any environment where it was not respected, and I have gained the strength to often refuse invitations whenever I have felt I would really enjoy being where I was more than going out. Take some time as soon as you can, for this is a very simple exercise.

Exercise

1. Start by saying to yourself things about yourself that you know are true—characteristics that you can describe as "I am_____." For example, "I am someone who loves trees." Now, if you don't love trees, don't say this, for you can't fool yourself. What is important here is to feel what you say, because the feeling is what lifts you emotionally, and that is the goal here. I want you to feel self-love, which is the root of health. I will give you a list of possibilities, and, even if you can feel only one of them is true, that is o.k. Do not judge yourself if you don't feel them all, for you are to focus on what is and not what is not. Schedule time for this exercise; for example, just as you are about to sleep, or just as you awake in the morning. Here is a short list, but do make up your own list, or add to this one if you like.

—I am someone who loves animals

(Allow time after making the affirmation for yourself to feel the powerful positive emotion that follows.)
—I am someone who loves rivers, lakes, the sea and mountains
—I am someone who loves children
—I am someone who loves the divine in my life
—I am someone who loves people (if that is hard, as it sometimes is for me, say "I am someone who loves the divine spirit in everyone else and that also lives in me.)
—I am someone who loves_____

Remember to take some time to do this. Make a commitment right now to take some time for this. It is best to do it when you can be quiet for five or ten minutes and let yourself feel the effect of focusing your powerful thoughts on what it is that is wonderful about you. Believe in yourself, for you cannot rely on another, or even hire someone to do that better than you can. Remember the word receptors? The cells in our bodies receive what we think. Thinking of all of what you are that lifts your feelings and brings you joy gives the gift of "healthy," or regenerative hormones and neurotransmitters to your cells. Think the best of yourself and you will grow deeply the roots of health in body, mind and emotion. Your own growth will be an example and an inspiration for a healthier world. Δ

REFERENCES

1. The information from Traynor-Kaplan is from a Spectrum International Radio interview. Spectrum: 1420 NW Gilman Blvd., Suite 2152, Issaquah, WA 98027. Interview tapes available for $9.95, plus $1 for post and handling.
2. See the excellent books *Head First: The Biology of Hope* (Dutton; $19.95) by Norman Cousins; *Who Gets Sick: Thinking and Health*, by Blair Justice, Ph.D. (Peak Press, 1987) and *Molecules of the Mind*, by Jon Franklin (Dell Publishing 1987), which all deal with the effects of neurotransmitters and molecular interactions in the brain/body. The Justice book explores more about how thoughts affect health, the Franklin work focuses upon chemical interactions and their effects on cells and therefore brain/body interfacing and Cousins' best-seller documents the most recent strides in mind-body research.
3. See the work of, among others, psychiatrist Eric Leskowitz, senior clinical instructor in psychiatry at Tufts University School of Medicine, who explores how specific mental events alter endocrine function and hormone secretion. *Theosophical Research Journal*, 5: 26-33.

Health is a consummation of a love affair of the body.

—Plato

Curing the Quantum Heart

Deepak Chopra, M.D.

WHEN PENICILLIN WAS DISCOVERED fifty years ago, it immediately began to cure disease. Infections that had killed patients for centuries were wiped out overnight, and whole hosts of bacteria were eliminated as a threat to human life. Sad to say, the same has not occurred with the discovery of mind-body medicine. We do not have a "mind-body penicillin." We do not have a major disease that has been defeated through the mind-body connection.

Why is that? The connection between mind and body is certainly as real as penicillin. Roughly one-third of all patients respond to the placebo effect, calling on their body's inner pharmacy to kill pain and combat illness. In theory, the mind can cure *any* disease. People have self-cured themselves of cancer, lupus, rheumatoid arthritis, and almost every other incurable illness. But the procedure remains unpredictable and evanescent. Every doctor has seen a tumor mysteriously regress in a breast-cancer patient, only to reappear in a matter of weeks or months. We all know that pain can be killed with a placebo pill, but we do not dare to perform surgery on that basis—the mind is still too changeable, fleeting and invisible to rely upon.

The technology that would rescue us from this dilemma does not exist on the level of either mind or body. We already comprehend that emotions can turn into molecules. Indeed, they must—fear in the mind is transformed into adrenaline in the body, and unless the adrenaline is produced, fear cannot have any physical effect. But the transformation itself is a huge paradox. In essence, mind is turning into matter, even though nothing could be further apart in nature's scheme than an emotion and a molecule. They live in entirely different worlds, and yet somehow, without any effort, each of us can bridge those worlds and cause them to interact.

We manage to do this, I believe, by bringing in a third element—the quantum. Having an emotion of fear is a quantum event, and so is producing a molecule of adrenaline. On the surface, this seems unbelievable, since molecules, emotions and quantum fluctuations appear completely unalike. But that is a mistake, born of the objective method. Inside a human being, the situation changes—whenever we think, feel or perceive through our five senses, we enter the quantum realm. Thinking is a quantum activity; it permits us to eavesdrop on the laws of nature that create the world.

Where can you stand objectively to watch an emotion turn into a molecule? Nowhere—you cannot see or touch an emotion; you can barely pin it down in time, and it has no home in space whatever; you cannot store it for future study, even though all emotions obviously reside in a mysterious storehouse called memory. Yet molecules can be objectively seen, stored and manipulated. They are easier to deal with than emotions, and therefore scientists always assume that the reality of molecules should be the benchmark, while the reality of emotions is somehow inferior.

Only in the quantum world does this situation change. A quantum event is also invisible, fleeting and unpredictable, just like our thoughts. Before the sun throws out light, where is it? Photons come out of nowhere and cannot be stored, except in that mysterious realm called the quantum field. They can barely be pinned down in time and have no home in space whatever, in that light occupies no volume and has no mass. At bottom, the quantum field is simply a creative source. It is empty of gross objects like hydrogen atoms and electrons, and yet without the quantum field as their background, these objects could not exist.

Similarly, without a quantum mechanical body, our physical bodies cannot exist. A physical body is not a lump of gross material—proteins, sugars, amines, peptides, etc.— which stand still in time and space. It is a constant flow of changing events. Its life and breath depend on transformations that can never cease. Seen in that light, the mind-body connection is not mysterious or unusual—it is the primary reality, compared to which all those lumps of protein and enzymes, even DNA itself, are secondary.

Emotions, molecules and quantum fluctuations are

not merely linked; they are the same. It is just our objective bias that calls them different. DNA is a fluctuation in the infinite, unbounded quantum field, and so is the thought, "I am happy." Fear and adrenaline are both identical quantum fluctuations. The reason you can put adrenaline into a bottle but not fear is simply due to our perceiving organs. Our eyes and fingers register quantum fluctuations as sight and touch; our minds register quantum fluctuations as emotions. But in the final analysis, "feeling" fear with your mind and "feeling" a drop of adrenaline with your heart is the same event viewed through different windows.

Without going into physics any deeper, let's just say that the quantum field is nature's creative source, and that we go there to create thoughts and emotions just as nature goes there to create matter and energy—the thought of a rose is just as quantum, therefore, as the creation of a star. If this is true, then it is easy to conceive of "quantum penicillin"—it would be whatever technique or therapy that puts us in touch with our quantum mechanical bodies, giving us control over the switching-station where mind turns into matter. Quantum penicillin cannot be touched or seen, nor is it a thought or emotion of any kind. It works by allowing us to be, not by manipulating our emotions but by allowing them to flow as nature intended them. Any disease could potentially be cured just by opening the channels that already connect mind, body and the quantum zone.

Quantum medicine does not even depend on our being human, for the quantum field is universal. Think about the following batch of rabbits. In the early 1970s, an Ohio State University research team was feeding some laboratory rabbits an extremely high-fat, high-cholesterol diet in order to measure the development of artery disease (atherosclerosis) induced by diet. As expected, the rabbits developed dangerous levels of serum cholesterol, followed by flagrant arterial lesions (fat-clogged arteries)—but there was one glaring exception. A single group of animals, fed the same diet as all the others, exhibited 60% less damage. The researchers were mystified, repeated their protocols, and again one batch of rabbits developed 60% less disease.

The mystery was solved in a most unexpected way: the graduate assistant assigned to one group of rabbits was found to be in the habit of taking them out of their cages and petting them tenderly before he fed them. It was this batch alone that withstood the toxic effects of their diet. Dr. Larry Dossey, who printed this fascinating story in his pioneering book, *Space, Time and Medicine* (New Science Library, 1982), comments: "Touching, petting, handling and gentle talking emerged as a crucial determinant in the disease process from which most of us will die: atherosclerosis." In other words, the rabbits' protection against massive doses of cholesterol was love.

This result flies in the face of the most cherished assumption in modern medicine, namely, that a disease which occurs on the molecular level must be fought on the molecular level. Love is not molecular, however. Not just rabbits, but humans respond to this obvious fact. One study of heart-attack survival conducted at Stanford in the early 1980s looked at some middle-aged men who had just been placed in an intensive cardiac care unit after suffering a coronary.

It is known that up to half of such patients will eventually die, usually in a matter of days or weeks, while others will survive, even when the amount of physical damage to the heart muscle appears to be the same. If damage to the heart does not correlate with survival, what does? According to this study, the best survivors were those men who thought their wives loved them; this psychological factor was a better predictor than any physical one, including the most sophisticated assessments via angiograms and EKGs of the condition of the heart itself. A man who felt loved might survive a massive coronary, while a lonely, unloved person might die of a relatively minor attack.

Love heals by the simplest means imaginable—it restores the channel that allows the mind to flow into the body via the quantum field. If you take a more complicated view, trying to analyze the millions of transformations that this involves, you are faced with potential chaos. A massive disease like coronary artery disease, which contributes to more than 75% of all heart attacks in the U.S., is the result of multiple influences in a person's life. Every thought contributes to the health of our hearts, because viewed from the quantum field, thoughts and heart cells are living the same life. Doctors who ignore this truth, who parlay a mere risk factor like cholesterol into something more, are misleading the public as well as themselves. Even on physical grounds they are mistaken, since thousands of people die of heart attacks every year who have "perfect" cholesterol. The reverse is also true: people with horrendous cholesterol levels live to advanced old age without suffering any heart problems.

Heart attacks are a human creation, an infliction

that modern man has brought upon himself. Nature did not create a heart disease germ or virus. She did not force us to eat foods that must damage our arteries ("primitive" peoples around the world have survived for thousands of years on extremely different diets, from the Eskimo's whale blubber to the native African's millet and sweet potatoes, and yet each diet sustains heart-attack rates that are a fraction of ours.) Rather than trying to shift the blame onto external forces, we need to look inside, at ourselves.

I do not think modern medicine has come to this conclusion fast enough, despite the hundreds of studies linking psychological factors with premature heart attacks. No one even mentioned these factors during my time in medical school in the late 1960s; today, mention is probably made, but the prejudice in favor of body over mind still runs strong. Interestingly, many patients seem to understand that their sick hearts indicate a deeper source of illness. The popular writer Michael Crichton was trained as a doctor at Harvard Medical School twenty-five years ago. He remembers the time he spent in the cardiac ward of a Boston teaching hospital. In their third and fourth years, all medical students spend a few months on a cardiac ward, but Crichton had a novel idea there. "I decided to learn something about the feelings the patients had about their disease," he writes. He was led to speculate that heart disease has a personal meaning for each individual.

What led him to think along this line were some famous pathology findings made in the early 1950s. During the Korean War autopsies were routinely performed on young soldiers who had been killed in battle, and doctors were surprised to find that the arteries of more than 70%

showed advanced stages of atherosclerosis; these young arteries were already building up fatty plaques, cutting oxygen off from the heart, and moving inexorably in the direction of a future heart attack.

Yet if men as young as seventeen had this disease, Crichton wondered, why did a typical male wait until his mid-forties or fifties before actually suffering a coronary? "You had to asume that all these patients had been walking around with clogged arteries since they were teenagers. A heart attack could happen any time.Why had they waited twenty or thirty years to develop a heart attack? Why had the heart attack happened this year and not next, this week and not last week?"

He decided on the unusual approach of going up to the patients and asking them point-blank why they had had a heart attack. He realized that his inquiries might set off unforeseeable reactions:

> My question "Why did you have a heart attack?" also implied that the patients had some choice in the matter, and therefore some control over their disease. I feared they might respond with anger. So I started with the most easygoing patient on the ward, a man in his forties who had had a mild attack.
> "Why did you have a heart attack?"
> "You really want to know?"
> "Yes, I do."
> "I got a promotion. The company wants me to move to Cincinnati. But my wife doesn't want to go. She has all her family here in Boston, and she doesn't want to go with me. That's why."

The man said this completely calmly, without any

sign of anger. When Crichton went on to question the rest of the ward, every other patient had a simlar answer:

> "My wife is talking about leaving me."
> "I didn't get the raise."
> "My wife wants another baby and I don't think we can afford it."

Not one person lacked an answer, yet not one mentioned arteriosclerosis as the cause of his heart attack or the standard risk factors, such as a high-fat diet, hypertension, lack of exercise and smoking. In the context of the late 1960s, when the mind-body connection was not considered quite legitimate, Crichton was perplexed by his patients' perspective. Now he looks back and writes,

> What I was seeing was that their explanations made sense from the standpoint of the whole organism, as a kind of physical acting-out. These patients were telling me stories of events that had affected their hearts in a metaphysical sense. They were telling me love stories. Sad love stories, which had pained their hearts. Their wives and families and bosses didn't care for them. Their hearts were attacked. And pretty soon, their hearts were literally attacked.

This perceptive account, taken from Crichton's latest book, *Travels* (Knopf, 1988), looks beyond the accepted framework of medicine into the quantum framework—instead of saying that these patients had metaphysical reasons for their heart attack, we could call them quantum reasons. It was not specific emotions or thoughts that triggered their disease, but a mere intention in awareness that underwent a quantum change, leaping the mind-body fence and turning into a heart attack.

The physical heart is not just part of the body; it is part of a person, and what the person knows, the heart knows. In the last ten years we have discovered various messenger molecules that can relay information from the brain to the heart—the hundreds of neurotransmitters and neuropeptides that have forced "hard" science to recognize the mind-body connection as something indisputably real. But new molecules don't really explain anything. At some level that exists outside physical limits, a sad thought becomes a sad heart, and if enough distorted thought patterns occur, a larger event occurs, in the form of distorted heart functions.

In 1988 a prominent article in the *New England Journal of Medicine* revealed that everyday situations, if embarrassing or distressing enough, do in fact cause coronaries on a miniature scale. Just by asking men to stand up and talk about themselves personally before a group of strangers, or making them multiply long numbers while being pressured to work faster, the researchers caused their subjects' hearts to go into the same convulsions that are characteristic of ischemic or "silent" heart attacks (those that damage the heart without causing noticeable pain). These miniature heart attacks may play a very big part in the prevalence of heart disease among people who think they are leading healthy lives.

What does all this diverse evidence mean? It means that the arena of heart disease is as large as our whole reality. When I examine a cardiac patient, I routinely take into account three distinct levels of his heart: the physical heart, the emotional heart and the "heart beyond the heart." Of the three, the last is by far the most important, because it escapes the limited confines of the body-mind and enters the unlimited region of the quantum field where all of us live, if only we realized it.

The physical and emotional planes are well covered in our present understanding already. Although it is unfortunately true that most cardiologists are fixated on the physical heart and rush to treat it with drugs and surgery, any well-informed patient can seek help for his emotional heart—getting at the source of negative beliefs, moods and emotional states is a recognized way of dealing with potential heart attacks. The Type As of this world can no longer delude themselves into thinking that their behavior is healthy. But once you spot a raging Type A personality, the process of deconditioning his anger, impatience, overweening drive and anxiety is no easy task. After all, it took a lifetime to instill these distorted emotional patterns, and they are not going to give way without intensive treatment (of the kind that most doctors and patients are not willing to undergo).

I feel that the real promise lies with the "heart beyond the heart." Before you can have Type A rage, you have to have something more basic—simple awareness. The mind, so full of thoughts and feelings, is built up from a foundation that is not full of thoughts; the mind is constantly moving, constantly spewing out reactions to life, but at the deepest level, it is still and silent. This is an age-old teaching we have learned to ignore; we may know that love averts heart disease, but we are at a total loss to engender love. Has any cardiologist turned a non-loving patient into a loving one?

Conventional medicine does not take us to this silent level of simple awareness, where love has its source in the quantum field. Therapy that goes beyond the mind works—for example, meditation has proved outstandingly successful in preventing heart disease. A 1987 study of 2,000 people using the TM, or Transcendental Meditation, technique showed that they were treated for heart disease 87% less often than the control group, which comprised more than 600,000 people of all ages and economic backgrounds.

This is a huge reduction. Anti-cholesterol drugs, which are rife with unpleasant side-effects, reduce heart disease by 30% at best, and to be successful with them requires extreme dedication to low-fat diet and a proper lifestyle. In the TM study conducted by research psychologist David Orme-Johnson and published in the journal *Psychosomatic Medicine*, no changes of lifestyle or diet was required. In and of itself, the continued practice of meditation made the "heart beyond the heart" healthy; in turn, the emotional heart became free of distorted patterns of thought and feeling; finally the physical heart derived the ultimate benefit.

The reason this approach worked is simple: if heart disease affects our entire reality, then treating one's entire reality, from the most basic level of awareness, should be most effective. Meditation is our first and best quantum medicine. Numerous papers have already shown that you can lower cholesterol and high blood pressure by meditating, but this study is unique in that it proved the final, holistic result—a large number of people who are not getting heart attacks. (Significantly, the best results were among meditators over the age of 65, although all age groups showed large improvements.)

In the light of this kind of finding, I have been practicing a new kind of medicine, called Maharishi Ayur-Veda, which takes all three levels of man, physical, mental and transcendent, into account, not just for heart disease but for all illness. Ayur-Veda had its origins in India more than 5,000 years ago; its Sanskrit name derives from two roots, *Ayus*, or life, and *Veda*, which means either "science" or "knowledge." Ayur-Veda therefore is the "science of life," an ancient tradition of health which was man's original "reality medicine"—it unites emotions, molecules and quantum fluctuations into a whole, instead of treating them as parts. In that way, Ayur-Veda is much truer to reality than our fragmented approach today, which puts too much on the objective side and leaves the subjective empty.

Today, mind-body medicine asumes that our deepest level must be mental or emotional, but Ayur-Veda disagrees. Behind both mind and body is the level of *Para*, which is Sanskrit for "beyond." There is a heart beyond the heart, a brain beyond the brain, an eye beyond the eye; all are united on the *para* level of the quantum field. By getting in contact with pure awareness, which is the only gateway to the *para* level, we also stand at the gateway of love.

This is what I tell my heart patients, at the same time that I tend to their physical and emotional problems. In the long run, it is their work on themselves that is going to nourish their hearts, not my brief attention. A few minutes of loving care is not going to change them. Yet non-loving patients can be turned into loving ones if you know how to go deep enough. Speak to the heart beyond the heart, educate them in meditation and Ayur-Veda, and the whole body understands. In brief, this is my rationale for the quantum medicine I practice. Once doctors learn the lessons of mind-body medicine, they are ready to take the next step. In the *para*, the beyond, is our real future. There we may fulfill the physician's deepest and best hope—a perfectly healthy patient living in a world freed from disease. Δ

There is a point of consciousness within everyone which has the seed of wholeness.
—*Dora Kunz*

The Hidden Dimensions of Health

Larry Dossey, M.D.

YOU CAN LEARN A LOT FROM FAIRY TALES. Take the story of King Midas, who wished that everything he touched turn to gold—and it did. Soon he was separated from those he loved, cut off from life. It was a prescription not only for fabulous wealth but for madness and death also, though in the beginning it seemed like only a formula for ecstasy. King Midas' experience, like most fairy tales, reminds us that there is an inner, esoteric, hidden aspect to events which, if ignored, can come back to haunt us.

We can imagine Midas' reasoning. If a little gold is good, an endless amount would be better, a fallacy he discovered too late.

It is the same in many areas of our own lives. A little potassium in the blood is good, but too much can kill. Love is also necessary, but it can smother and kill. Water is necessary for life, but only in the right amount; if drunk to excess it can kill like cyanide.

What about health? Can it too be toxic? Can we have too much of it, like Midas' gold? The question is serious. Today it is taken for granted that the more health the better. But is there an esoteric side to health that suggests otherwise?

This question is particularly relevant in the New Age, when we are assured on every hand that we "create our own reality," including health and illness. But what if there is some hidden calculus to health, some "range of normal" below or above which "health," like potassium and the water content of the body is toxic? In certain situations, would it be wise to "lower" health, just as we might want to reduce the blood's potassium level if it is too high?

We call these "health-lowering" experiences "illness and disease." Sometimes, as strange as it may seem, they give us just what we need. They can bring us into balance or increase our wisdom and understanding; they can eventually lead, paradoxically, to greater health—all in spite of the fact that we may not know this at the time.

In fact, our bodies require illness—little micro-challenges of disease—in order to be healthy. That's the way our immune system develops. By being repeatedly clobbered early in life by a variety of viruses, bacteria, fungi and innumerable foreign agents, we develop the capacity to resist them. Without these mini-diseases health would never happen and death would be certain. In medical practice we put this principle to work by re-creating it whenever we give immunizations and vaccines.

But what if our body and mind protested when challenged with these illnesses by saying, "My birthright is to be healthy. Since I create my own reality by the choices I make, my choice is health, not these endless harrassments by this army of microorganisms." The result would not be health but certain death. Sometimes the body does actually say no to these challenges because it can't muster an immune response to them because of inborn defects, and the result is the "bubble babies" who must live in constant isolation and who usually die from infection at an early age.

Fortunately we do not have to think about these complex processes; they occur below the level of our awareness during the early years of life. But trouble can come later when we try to completely control our health from conscious awareness by taking a "the more the better" approach, just as King Midas did. This has become epitomized in the "you create your own reality" philosophy of the New Age, in which one tries to sculpt a reality that contains a minimum of discomfort. The formula invoked is a simple one. In column number one go the desireable experiences such as vitality, longevity, happiness, a lovely body etc. In column number two go pain, suffering, illness, disability, death etc. "Creating our own reality" is equated with making the "right choices"—the decisions that bring about only the events in column number one.

On a certain level it is very true that we do create our own health-reality. If we realize that smoking causes cancer, emphysema and heart disease, the choice to not smoke is an active step toward health. Endless examples of this sort could be given. Social isolation, for example, is related to higher death rates from a broad variety of diseases, so that a choice of noninvolvement with the world is a choice, conscious or otherwise, leading toward illness. The idea that behaviors, attitudes, emotions and feeling states enter into bodily health is no longer a matter of debate. As evidence, the developing field of psychoneuroimmunology clearly demonstrates the unity and interrelatedness of the mind and the immune and neurological systems.

This domain of health I want to call *rational* because it is structured according to the dictates of reason. In the area of rational health, values follow common sense—health and longevity are good; pain, suffering and death are bad, etc. This perspective of health is solidly embedded in a particular world view we seldom question—flowing, linear, one-way time ("a long life is better than a short one"), causality ("smoking causes cancer"), and an objective world that is "out there." In sum, this is the foundation of beliefs we invoke when we try to create better health through making the right choices.

But in addition to rational healing there is another region that could be called *paradoxical* healing. A paradox is an event or experience that appears false or absurd, but which in fact may be true. With reason, what you see or do is what you get; but with paradox, what you get is unexpected and is frequently what you *don't* see or do. Here another world view comes into play that creates and sustains paradox. This world view no longer conforms to common sense. In it, time is no longer linear, and events don't happen serially but simply "are." Causality, too, is different; cause and effect are not strung out like a row of dominoes, one event following from another, but exist as a totality and unity.

This view of reality is the foundation of an indivisible unity of all things and events in which absolutes like "good" and "bad" become entirely relative.

A curious result is that in the paradoxical domain there is no such distinction as "good" and "bad" health. Neither is a long life necessarily better than a short one. Pain and suffering are similarly seen as an integral part of pleasure and happiness. In fact, in the paradoxical domain *all* opposites are unified as a single whole, both necessary for their mutual existence. Like light and shadow, husband and wife, or the two sides of a coin, they define each other. *None* of which makes sense when viewed from the perspective of rational healing.

The entire question of whether or not we create our own health-reality by the choices we make becomes a nonquestion in the paradoxical domain. As Jehangir Chubb, former professor of philosophy at the University of Bombay, put it,

> One does not choose. ...[We do] not... make a list of things that we have to hold onto or discard.... One doesn't start by discriminating between things one regards as good and those which one regards as evil, and eliminating the latter. One starts with what one is. And if we find that there is any relationship which is helpful, which brings about peace and harmony and satisfaction, that's all to the good. ...It's not a question of giving up something, but straightening oneself out. ...It should come spontaneously; [one] doesn't set out to eliminate something by using the surgeon's knife."[1] One is reminded of the ancient Zen saying: "The making of distinctions is the sickness of the mind."

A frequent objection to this point of view is that it is too passive. It condones inactivity and nonaction, letting the world wash over us as it will. It thus *dis*empowers people who might otherwise choose to improve their health, while the thrust of the New Age is to *em*power them. But while this objection seems reasonable to the rational mind, it is untrue in the domain of paradoxical healing. In fact, one is not mired in inactivity in *either* domain, even that of paradox; even in it one can act with *enormous* energy and decisiveness. It is only that the premises from which one acts in the region of paradox are different than in the rational domain—there is a different sense of time and causation; a diminished sense of urgency and desperation; an abiding sense of unity and wholeness; and a different concept of self, as we shall see.

In many if not most New Age circles, physical health and spiritual health are linked together and often equated. Spiritual awareness leads to physical harmony according to this view. Many persons find evidence for this in their own lives. When they take up meditation, e.g., physical ailments may indeed disappear, vitality and energy levels may increase, and one may feel more alive than ever before. Empirical studies confirm these impressions. Persons who pursue certain meditation programs *are* healthier, they visit doctors less frequently and they spend far less on health care. The tendency, therefore, is to say that if a *little* spiritual growth leads to an increase in health, a *lot* of spiritual awareness will result in even more health, possibly physical perfection. But again, while this conclusion seems perfectly logical in the domain of reason, it breaks down in the higher regions of paradox. It is easy to confirm this. As Ken Wilber, the transpersonal psychologist, has pointed out, three of the most spiritually advanced persons of this century have died of cancer—J. Krishnamurti (cancer of the pancreas), Suzuki Roshi (cancer of the stomach) and Ramana Maharshi (cancer of the stomach). The case of Ramana Maharshi, one of India's most beloved modern saints, is particularly instructive. During his final days and weeks his suffering was almost unbearable. His devotees were frequently awakened by his screams of pain during the night. For them it was an enormous ordeal. They could not understand why such a saintly person, their spiritual teacher, would have fallen prey to cancer in the first place, and why he should have to suffer so. By morning Maharshi's pain would frequently abate, whereupon he would remind them that his true Self was not a function of his body. Even though his body could sicken, suffer and die, his larger Self remained perfect and incorruptible.

If there is no one-to-one correlation between spiritual and physical health for such God-realized mystics, how much less for anyone else?

Ramana Maharshi was suggesting to his devotees that it is possible to be completely healthy on one level and fatally ill on another. This implies that there are different levels of wellness, therapy and healing, each with different rules and dynamics that govern them. Lumping them all together creates great confusion. An awareness of these different modes can help us understand how healing operates—or does not operate—in our own efforts to be healthy.

We can divide these modes of healing into different "eras." Era I medicine is the commonest type of healing practiced today in cosmopolitan societies. It is scientific, allopathic, Newtonian, "modern" medicine. It has its roots in empirical science and operates on the classical world view that applies to rational healing described above. According to its tenets, all disease is physical and originates in the body because of the malfunction of atoms or molecules deep within the body. In Era I medicine there is no place for the mind, which is viewed simply as an expression of the biochemistry of the brain.

Era II medicine, which can be called "mind-body" medicine, is different. It recognizes consciousness as a causal factor in health and illness, and accepts a two-way relationship linking the mental and the physical. Era II medicine became very prominent when psychosomatic phenomena were described in great detail, particularly in the period following World War II. It is still gathering steam with the development of new disciplines such as psychoneuroimmunology, mentioned above. Era II healing events are quite commonly described by advocates of the self-created health movement. These are basically intra-body processes that clearly show the capacity of human consciousness to bring about healing effects in the physical organism. But Era II healing, like Era I, is still solidly anchored in the rational domain, employing the same classical world view.

Many New Age enthusiasts believe Era II medicine is the highest level that healing can attain, for it recognizes the ability of human consciousness to change the physical body. But there is yet another, higher level—Era III medicine—that lies beyond it.

Era III medicine is the domain of paradoxical healing described above. Strictly speaking it is not an "era" at all, for it lies outside time. Not only is it timeless, it also differs from Eras I and II by being acausal, unpredictable and nonlinear. This means that cause A may sometimes lead to effect B, sometimes not. Put another way, the results that one observes are not predictable from initial conditions—which is why this form of medicine and healing can seem highly paradoxical. It is also why some highly spiritual persons enjoy perfect physical health, and why others, as mentioned above, do not. It may also account in part for why many reprobates and spiritually degenerate persons live long lives in peak physical condition.

Era III medicine invokes a view of consciousness unlike the other eras. In them, consciousness is "local"— i.e., it is confined to the person's body and brain (localization in space) and to the present moment (localization in time). This is why healing seems to be a genuinely local, intra-body experience when consciousness is involved in Era II (mind-body) medicine. But Era III is the domain of *nonlocal* mind, and thus *nonlocal* healing. Why nonlocal? Because it recognizes that consciousness is not confined, limited or localized to points in space such as brains or bodies, or to points in time such as the present moment or even single lifetimes. This means that consciousness is *unbounded*—and if unbounded, then unitary and One. There is thus never any question of self-created health or illness in Era III medicine, for there is fundamentally no individual self or mind who could do the creating—only the larger Self that contains all the lesser, individual selves.

Era III medicine recognizes an inner divinity of all

persons because of the nonlocal qualities possessed by all minds. For to be nonlocal or unbounded in space is to be omnipresent, and to be nonlocal or unbounded in time is to be infinite, eternal and immortal. Omnipresence and eternality are attributes of God, we have always maintained; but with the recognition of our nonlocal nature they become *our* qualities as well. This inner divinity has been described by the mystics of all the great traditions. Examples include the Hindu aphorism from the Upanishads, "*tat tvam asi*" (thou art that), and the words of Jesus in John 10:34, ". . . you are gods."

Perhaps the *most* paradoxical aspect of Era III healing is that, ultimately, there is nothing that *needs* healing. How could there be? How could something eternal, infinite and immortal be improved upon? How could something unified, whole and complete be made *more* complete? The great mystics know this and state it unequivocally—even visionaries such as Ramana Maharshi who die of horrible illnesses, as we saw above.

The nonlocal consciousness recognized in Era III medicine is not a fantasy; it is the way our consciousness actually behaves. Empirical evidence amply demonstrates this. Nonlocal effects of consciousness have surfaced in experiments dealing with the effects of prayer in coronary care units of modern hospitals. Doctor Randolph Byrd at San Francisco General Hospital has demonstrated, in a prospective, controlled, double-blind study of almost four hundred patients, that prayer results in powerful therapeutic effects *at a great distance*.[2] Similar effects are seen in the experiments of Professor Robert G. Jahn and Brenda J. Dunne at Princeton University's Engineering Anomalies

Research Laboratory, which deal with the ability of minds to share information even when separated by up to six thousand miles. The results of both of these experiments can best be explained by a nonlocal model of human consciousness. In the Jahn-Dunne experiments, in which information is mentally conveyed by a "sender" to a "receiver," in most cases the receiver actually "gets" the message up to three days before it is sent, implying nonlocality of the mind in time as well as in space.[3] Space does not permit a detailed discussion of these and other studies that are relevant to the nonlocal nature of human consciousness. Anyone wanting to explore this area may read my *Recovering the Soul* in which this evidence is reviewed.[4]

Although there is no imperative for healing (because of the completeness, unity and perfection inherent in the domain of Era III medicine), healing nonetheless does occur spectacularly in this paradoxical region. In fact, Era III medicine is the domain not only of the remarkable effects of prayer, as mentioned, but of miraculous and ;unexplainable healing events as well. This is where the unpredictable may happen—where terminal, fatal diseases vanish and where "spontaneous remissions" occur.

The key to understanding Era III medicine and paradoxical healing in general is the nonlocal nature of human consciousness—mind that is outside time and space and the individual person. This means there is a larger Self that includes all individual selves and which is Divine—and thus all-powerful. And if it is omnipotent, "miracles" should be *expected* and should never be a cause for surprise when they occur. But we should always realize that healing events in this domain are *always* superfluous; for as we noted, what is already whole cannot be made *more* whole. In this sense paradoxical healing, when it comes, always seems to be a matter of grace—a blessing, a gift from the Universe.

There are vast implications of nonlocal mind for both patients and healers. For patients, illness is no longer a solitary event because of the absorption of all single minds into the One Mind. Illness thus becomes a shared experience. This can be a source of profound comfort during illness, which frequently generates a sense of isolation from the larger community of the healthy. The recognition of nonlocal mind can also assist healers by connecting them with all therapists past, present and future. This is the equivalent of summoning millions of consultants on any given case—shamans and folk-healers from ages past, and specialists who exist in the present and who are yet to be. Similarly for patients, having access to the collective wisdom of the One Mind can assist us when our personal wisdom fails.

I believe this fount of strength and wisdom is appallingly overlooked in the New Age, when so much responsibility for health-creation and right-choosing seems to have been assigned to the individual. I find it both curious and sad that many persons feel compelled to dwell persistently in individuality, cutting themselves off from this collective wisdom and power. They do not seem to realize that relinquishing the hold of the ego and the solitary "I" leads to *more* power, not less.

In order to emphasize this available source of

empowerment and comfort, I want to quote three persons of vastly different backgrounds, who make essentially the same point. The first is Aldous Huxley, who wrote so brilliantly about the perennial philosophy, the common esoteric thread running through the world's mystical traditions. He said,

> Total awareness . . . reveals . . . that I am profoundly ignorant, that I am impotent to the point of helplessness and that the most valuable elements in my personality are unknown qualities . . . yet, somehow or other, here I am, but alive and kicking.... I can only infer that the no-I, which looks after my body and gives me my best ideas, must be amazingly intelligent, knowledgeable and strong.[5]

Next, an unlikely source, a modern physicist—Erwin Schrodinger, whose wave equations lie at the heart of modern quantum physics:

> Thus you can throw yourself flat on the ground, stretch out on Mother Earth, with the certain conviction that you are one with her and she with you. You are as firmly established, as invulnerable as she, indeed a thousand times more invulnerable. As surely as she will engulf you tomorrow, so surely will she bring you forth anew to new striving and suffering. And not merely "some day": now, today, every day she is bringing you forth, not *once* but thousands of times, just as every day she engulfs you a thousand times over. For eternally and always there is only *now*, one and the same now; the present is the only thing that has no end.[6]

And an observation from one of the most astute figures in the New Age movement, psychologist and writer Patricia Sun, who vividly describes the potency and importance of paradox in healing:

> The thing in the New Age now is to talk about how "you created it." It gets a little annoying...[because] there's something missing there....you are an effect of this universe and...you are completely in response to it, receptive to it.

> As you paradoxically let yourself be empty and say, "I don't know," you make a wonderful space to be filled, and as you are filled you expand and you are greater . . . . You win by simultaneously knowing you are a pipsqueak in the universe, you don't know anything. . . . The minute you realize the paradox inherent in our perception of the universe, you will have broadened your ability to perceive the universe.[7]

These three points of view may strike many who are interested in employing their own consciousness in improving their health as too passive and disempowering, because the healing they describe takes place outside our conscious awareness, unassisted by our own efforts. Yet there is *always* an element of initiative and effort that is required, even in paradoxical, Era III medicine. Even those who experience miracle cures such as at Lourdes must *go* to the shrine; it does not come to them. Yet it cannot be emphasized too strongly that Era III medicine or paradoxical healing is overwhelmingly a mode of *being*, not of *doing*. It requires attunement and alignment more than active effort. If this strategy seems too passive, perhaps that is only because we have become obsessed with the aggressive, masculine, "yang" part of ourselves, and have become overreliant not only on *doing* but on *things*—whether drugs or surgery, or herbs, crystals or the other accoutrements that have become commonplace in many healing circles.

One of our most difficult tasks is giving up the

incessant need always to *control* our health. Indeed, self-control and self-creation have become the credo of much of the New Age health movement. But in the regions of paradox, control cannot be achieved; here we simply cannot bring the Universe into compliance by clobbering it with reason or effort. In the paradoxical domain, events seem to happen out of the blue, as if uncaused—again, the Universe's gift to us. Our greatest task is to set the stage for these events, to facilitate their occurrence, as many mystics, visionaries and poets learn to do. This means learning to cooperate with the world, not controlling it. If this seems like an unkind, stubborn or foreign way for the Universe to behave, it helps to recall that many other healing events also follow this pattern, of which everyone is aware. One of the commonest is psychological healing. When the psyche repairs itself in the process of psychoanalysis, we often speak of unexpected "breakthroughs" that happen out of the blue. The brilliant Scottish psychiatrist R.D. Laing has described this process as follows, which is a perfect description of *any* healing even in the paradoxical domain:

> The really decisive moments in psychotherapy, as every patient or therapist who has ever experienced them knows, are unpredictable, unique, unforgettable, always unrepeatable and often indescribable.[8]

Emptiness, watching, waiting and silence can be a forerunner and precondition of some of the most powerful healing events we can possibly experience. The Pulitzer Prize-winning poet Gary Snyder tells of an incident from history that dramatically illustrates these points. Alvar Nunez Cabeza de Vaca, the great Spanish explorer who followed Columbus' wake to the new world, was shipwrecked on the Texas coast and was beset by the hostile natives living there. He took refuge where he could find it, including a pit in the harsh Texas territory where he spent several winter nights sleeping naked under a north wind. Yet he survived, and then he discovered that a wondrous event had happened: He had the power to heal. Thus on his way westward across the continent he would heal sick native people along the way as his fame spread ahead of him. Eventually de Vaca made his way back to Mexico and became once again a civilized Spaniard. At this point the events seemed to reverse themselves. Drawing closer to civilization he lost not only the ability to heal but the will to heal as well. As he said, there were "real doctors" in the city, and as he came nearer to them he began to doubt his own healing powers.

De Vaca's ability to heal was preceded by a profound emptiness, a shipwreck of both body and spirit, a dark night of the soul in which he did not know he would survive. Through it he became connected to something higher and larger than himself—which meant that the emptiness he experienced was not really a void at all but a state that was immensely empowering. And as he gradually became filled up again by the expectations and pressures of reentering civilization, his emptiness—and power—vanished.

It is the same for many patients who undergo radical, life-changing healing. They frequently describe a state in which they accept the universe on its own terms, not dictating what ought or should happen. This experiential state is connected to yet another paradox, again described by poet Gary Snyder:

> To be truly free one must take on the basic conditions as

they are: painful, impermanent, and imperfect; and then be grateful, for in a fixed universe there would be no freedom.[9]

The points I have tried to make in this brief article have been hard for me to learn as a physician. Like most modern doctors I was trained to be a doer, an interventionist. Through my own experience I know that many persons, in their enthusiasm for applying their own powers of consciousness to their health, are easily swept up in the same aggressive, active stance as we physicians, although their aggressiveness is manifested in different ways.

Consequently I believe a bit of genuine reflection is in order. The past decade has been a heady one for New Agers interested in what the mind can do. Untapped inner potentials have been discovered, and new body-mind connections seem to roll out of scientific laboratories every day. Clearly, consciousness is back on the table in medicine. But let us guard against oversimplifying what "consciousness" and "healing" mean. And in our enthusiasm to harness the mind on behalf of the body, let us focus on the *whole* picture of the mind, not part of it. Let us acknkowledge, too, that there may be aspects of the world that simply do not exist for us to harness; and that what we *cannot* do can be as important and empowering as what we *can* do.

This plea is, of course, nothing new. The hidden, powerful, paradoxical dimensions of existence have been glimpsed by our greatest visionaries for millenia. These are quintessentially visions of unity—an awareness that everything, including health and ilness, birth and death, light and shadow, form ultimately an indissoluble whole.

91

In closing, let us catch a glimpse of this vision through a sublime passage from Hermann Hesse's *Siddhartha:*

> Siddhartha listened... completely absorbed, quite empty, taking in everything.... He had often heard all this before ... but today they sounded different. He could no longer distinguish the different voices—the merry voice from the weeping voice, the childish voice from the manly voice. They all belonged to each other: the lament of those who yearn, the laughter of the wise, the cry of indignation and groan of the dying. They were all interwoven and interlocked, entwined in a thousand ways. And all the voices, all the goals, all the yearnings, all the sorrows, all the pleasures, all the good and evil, all of them together was the world. All of them together was the stream of events, the music of life. When Siddhartha listened attentively . . . when he did not listen to the sorrow or laughter, when he did not blind his soul to any one particular voice... but heard them all, the whole, the unity; then the great song of a thousand voices consisted of one word: *Om.* Δ

REFERENCES
1. "The Silent Mind: Interview with Jehangir Chubb," in *A Bell Ringing in the Empty Sky: The Best of the Sun*, vol. II, Sy Safransky, ed. (San Diego: Mho and Mho Works, 1987), pp 161-186.
2. Randolph G. Byrd, "Positive Effects of Intercessory Prayer in a Coronary Care Unit Population," *Southern Medical Journal*, vol. 81, no. 7, July 1988, pp. 826-829.
3. Robert G. Jahn and Brenda J. Dunne, *Margins of Reality* (New York: Harcourt Brace Jovanovich, 1987).
4. Larry Dossey, *Recovering the Soul: A Scientific and Spiritual Search* (New York: Bantam, 1989).

5. Aldous Huxley, *Tomorrow and Tomorrow and Tomorrow* (New York: New American Library, 1964), p. 54.

6. Erwin Schrodinger, *My View of the World* (Woodbridge, CT: Ox Bow Edition, 1983), p. 22.

7. Elizabeth Rose Campbell, "Patricia Sun," in *A Bell Ringing in the Empty Sky: The Best of the Sun*, vol. 1, Sy Safransky, ed. (San Diego: Mho and Mho Works, 1985), pp. 269-270.

8. R.D. Laing quoted in Fritjof Capra, *Uncommon Wisdom* (New York: Simon and Schuster, 1988), p. 116.

9. Gary Snyder, "The Etiquette of Freedom," *Sierra* vol. 74, no. 5, Sept.-Oct. 1989, p. 75 ff.

10. Hermann Hesse, *Siddhartha* (New York: New Directions, 1957), pp. 137-138.

Nothing in this world remains unchanged but for one moment only. Everything changes aspect. It dissolves, merges with other elements and displays a new aspect, different from the previous one.

—Heraclitus

Surviving
Life-Threatening Illness
An Interview with Jeanne Segal, Ph.D.

Scott Miners: You described in your book *Living Beyond Fear: Coping with the Emotional Aspects of Life-Threatening Illness* the transformational abilities of a person who is critically ill. What are the transformational abilities?

Jeanne Segal: The most obvious is a tremendous motivation to live. A desire that is so strong it enables individuals to confront their deepest fears. Critically ill people can rapidly mobilize to address sources of chronic stress and depression that have plagued their lives for years.

Illness also helps us to become aware of our priorities. In this context it is not uncommon for people to begin making very different choices. For example, they begin to take time for self-understanding and self-development. They want to participate in activities that genuinely feel rewarding and often find that they now have the time to reach out and become involved with other people. Of

---

course, all of this takes time, which ironically becomes available when one's life is threatened.

S.M.: These folks really won't take time for themselves unless it becomes very obvious that they need to.

J.S.: Right—crisis gives people permission to take time for themselves. A health crisis also gives them permission to take themselves and life seriously. Another irony here is that when people do this they find themselves lightening up. The quality of life is what counts the most, and a lot of heavy things that used to seem important lose their grip on us. This also explains why some people are able to become risk takers for the first time in their lives. They are willing, in that moment of desperation, to try something new, to take risks.

S.M.: What do people who successfully gothrough a critical illness do to get themselves through it?

J.S.: Superficially they appear to tap internal and external resources that strengthen and motivate them. The "will to live" or the "faith that is found" appears to be the tether that pulls a person through a critical illness. But if you ask the question "Exactly where is this will or faith found?" you get a very surprising answer. It lies in individuals' capacity to perceive and act on physical and emotional feelings that generate from within their own bodies.

It takes more than thought to motivate and sustain us throughout a crisis. It also requires the sources of energy and inspiration, wisdom that can be tapped by paying very careful attention to the body and the messages it constantly sends. In order to really pay attention to the body, one must tune in to what is going on inside: physically, emotionally and intuitively.

S.M.: So they're becoming more aware of their bodies and their feelings?

J.S.: Feelings are mostly in the body below the bridge of the nose. The only feeling you have in your head is a headache. So they learn to let go or their thought processes for at least a little while. It isn't that they stop thinking or become anti-intellectual, but they become more than just thinkers. They focus on all their feelings, including physical sensations and all emotions—sadness and fear, but also joy and love.

S.M.: How do they do that? What are some of the ways that you have experienced that they do that?

J.S.: Feeling our feelings is something that we all did at one time. If we had a little stomach pain we knew it. If we sensed danger we were aware; and if we felt happy or sad, we were intensely conscious of what we felt. Infants and young children do this naturally and intuitively. Every time we breathe deeply we intensify our feelings, but as we "mature" we begin to distance ourselves from them. We go to school where we're told to sit still at desks all day long. In order not to cry and scream out we learn to hold our breath and squeeze our bodies.

The maturing process often takes us further and further away from our feelings as we get better at hiding our vulnerability—even from ourselves! So much in our culture unfortunately encourages this kind of behavior. We are taught that emotions are childish and that thinking is superior to feeling. Unfortunately when we shut out the vulnerable feelings we also shut out positive feeling. This is the source of the apathy and depression that so many experience.

S.M.: So one way for people to be successful is to get out of that cycle of denying their feelings because they've learned it from our society in some way, and come around full cycle to recognize their feelings again?

J.S.: Yes! But that is not an easy thing for most people to do. After years of avoiding difficult emotions, getting comfortable with feeling may take some practice. Survivors intuitively give themselves permission to experience their feelings, but anyone who is strongly motivated can relearn what this means. People can and must become aware of their internal environment. It is the source that guides and informs their healing process. As I said, survivors intuitively turn inward for sources of strength and motivation.

S.M.: They get their own answers. They love themselves enough to get answers or to take the time to themselves they need for evaluation.

J.S.: Hmmm, let's examine what it means to really love yourself. To truly love myself I have to be able to look at the whole of me and feel accepting of it—including the parts that are far less than perfect. If love means to notice and to acknowledge all my good parts and to avoid the parts that I may think are less than perfect, I don't call that a very quality love.

S.M.: It's rather loving yourself enough to acknowledge that you have fears or angers and still maintain you self-esteem.

J.S.: Yes! If I feel loved or if you feel loved, it's because we feel that the person knows the whole—everything about us. If all they look at is the pretty exterior then it somehow doesn't feel the same as if a person tells you they love you and they know you through and through. Self-love works the same way. It's very hard to have deep self-love without self-awareness.

S.M.: And the more that you become self-aware, it seems then, it becomes more of a challenge, you have more of an adventure.

J.S.: Indeed, the more opportunity you have to know, the greater the opportunity to love. However, while self-awareness allows us to become more self accepting, self-knowledge doesn't *guarantee* self-acceptance. Some people will become self-aware and then judge or criticize what they find. That's obviously not going to improve their self-love. Judgment and criticism can keep self-awareness from becoming self-understanding and self-love. Compassion for ourselves along with a good sense of humor can go a long way in helping to offset judgment and criticism.

S.M.: So are awareness and acknowledgement and maintaining self-esteem and humor and basic care for self the bottom line for successful people?

J.S.: Awareness, acceptance and the ability to really process your physical and emotional feelings in a healthy and appropriate way. When people feel overwhelmed or out of control, their self-esteem is undermined.

S.M.: What about self-judgment. How does that affect health?

J.S.: Judgment is an exhausting and stressful process. It's often what we do instead of dealing with the things that hurt us, or frighten or anger us. We get into our heads with lists of judgments and thus escape from what needs to be done. We escape from the experience of our feelings. That kind of process is also negative because it takes you away from the work that you really need to be doing. It sucks up your energy and cripples your will to live. But there's nothing about feeling intense grief or intense anger or intense fear, at the feeling level, that in any undermines your health. As far as the body is concerned, a feeling is a feeling is a feeling, and it's all okay.

Pushing away feeling, numbing running away from what we feel by intellectualizing emotions or acting out shuts down immune functioning.

S.M.: If you could pick one person out of all the people whom you have worked with, which case would best demonstrate these qualities of survival, of health?

J.S.: The qualities I've been talking about are characteristic of survivors. I'm fortunate to have worked with many people who started out fearful and overwhelmed but were also motivated to do whatever it took to increase their chance for survival.

S.M.: What about someone who had the greatest life-threatening illness?

J.S.: I've worked with many individuals who've had an incredibly bleak prognosis. Fifteen years ago someone with cancer of the lungs or brain was automatically given a death sentence as many with H.I.V. infection are today. Some of those people are alive today. I see them on the streets of the city I live in. Survival has been my life's work. I've been drawn to people who have not given up on themselves, though everyone else has given up on them.

S.M.: In other words, they've been to the doctors, to the hospitals, and everyone has said, "I'm sorry, I can't help you."

J.S.: Often that has been the case. I've been fascinated by survival because survivors are willing to do things differently in order to live.

S.M.: So you work with people who are at the end of their ropes, and ready to do just about anything. You say to them, "I think you've got some feelings here that you're not facing." And in your work you say probably the most commonly disregarded feeling is fear.

J.S.: The feeling that is first perceived is more likely to be sadness or grief, but as you work with sadness and grief, you get to a deep sense of fear that is usually connected with despair, hopelessness or helplessness. That's often how it runs its course.

S.M.: Is the fear "I'm not good enough, I won't make it?"

101

J.S.: The deepest fear is that I can't do anything about this anyway. The situation is hopeless and I'm hopeless—life is hopeless. Despair stemming from fear surfaces as grief, rage and depression.

S.M.: That is suffering.

J.S.: And it undermines the will to live. When you feel hopeless and helpless about some situation in your life, whether it's conscious or unconscious, it affects immune response as well as quality of life. You believe in a deep, deep way that there is nothing that can be done and this despair undermines the will to live and sends a shut down message to your immune system.

S.M.: So what is the first step in your work then, after you find a person who may have come in their own perception to the seeming end?

J.S.: They're dissatisfied with whatever resources they're familiar with, but at the same time there is some spark, some interest in continuing to explore life and new possibilities. Some people don't have that interest. They really are consciously ready and willing to die, and I don't believe that it is my place to try and change such decisions. I support these people in having quick and painless deaths. Those individuals who have not been completely wasted by their illness and still have some strength left have a choice. Those I work with are willing to address their despair and all the things that frighten and overwhelm them. They ask, "What is my despair about? Do I really believe that I can never be loved or useful? Do I really believe that I will never be capable of loving or making a contribution," etc? People have different things that they feel hopeless and helpless about. But if they can start to face their fear and despair, they find that there are alternatives and with this awareness comes "the will to live." Transformation at the practical level means you change things in your life in a very substantive way so that you can extend and add greater meaning and purpose to your life.

S.M.: Say I come to you with AIDS and I've tried everything and I don't seem to be healing, and I haven't given up hope. I've just given up on medical cures, drugs, and everything else, and I hear about you.

J.S.: I don't want to imply that the people I see do not see medical doctors. Most who see me will still be continuing with some kind of treatement. But they will also be sufficiently self-aware to know there is more they need to do to recover. They'll come into an H.I.V. positive group and they'll begin working with the understanding that if they're blocked emotionally, this isn't good for controlling H.I.V. disease. In order to get the maximum effect with whatever medications, diet, or regimen they're doing—their emotional coping skills need to be will developed. Whatever positive things they may be doing for themselves can and will be offset by emotional stress, depression, fear, consuming rage or sadness. They must learn how to cope with these feelings in ways that don't drain and exhaust them.

This, as I have said, is not a very popular thing to do. Emotional awareness is feared and desecreated. Moreover, emotional awareness is especially difficult for the gay population, because feelings were so painful for so many.

S.M.: They feel discriminated against.

J.S.: They feel discriminated against, misunderstood, maligned, ignored and rejected. For many gays their teenage years were especially hurtful because they had feelings that they themselves often didn't understand. Nor was there anyone to talk to or support them at this time. If they have not already done so, many, many people then make the choice to cut off emotional awareness.

S.M.: That's the point where self-judgment begins, and it's reinforced by the judgment of society.

J.S.: Exactly. And then this process takes a tremendous amount of your life-force, of your energy, to not feel what's going on, especially if the feelings are intense and there is a lot of justification for frustration, anger, hurt, sadness and fear.

S.M.: What is your advice or what would you like to tell people in the health professions who work with life-threatened people—something we all seem to face.

J.S.: The most important thing is to get in touch with your own fears. To work well you have to have faced these issues yourself. If you're going to work with people's fear of death, you had better look at the possibility of your own death and the death of your loved ones. You've got to be authentic in order to help people in this way. If you're a person who's going to be asking the most emotionally-charged and intimate kinds of questions, you had better damn-well be authentic. You have to be able to handle such questions yourself.

You have to have had some transformational experiences yourself in order to be of help to another who is going through something. I've looked carefully and in depth at my own perceptions of death and dying. Where H.I.V. disease is concerned, one also has to have a great deal of security and comfort with one's own sexuality. I think that's one of the reasons that makes H.I.V. disease especially difficult for health professionals. It's tough working with cancer and other life-threatening diseases, but with H.I.V. there's an additional charge, particularly when male doctors are concerned. Many people have a real discomfort around their own sexuality that interferes with their capacity to be compassionately present with a gay man.

S.M.: What keeps you going, what's the inspiration in your life?

J.S.: I desire a sense of fulfillment and satisfaction from being helpful to people. And I can see the positive results of what I'm able to help people do for themselves. I get great satisfaction, and a sense of purpose from feeling that I am genuinely of service, and helpful to others. I believe that what I do does make a difference. It's demanding work, but many of the people who I work with reward me by teaching me about life and hope, courage and faith. I feel very privileged to be doing the work I am doing. Δ

Self-Talk and Feeling-Interactive Affirmations

PERHAPS ONE OF THE MOST POWERFUL and simple ways to change one's health for the better is through the intentional and focused use of creative self talk—talk of an affirmative nature, talk that enhances one's life. This is more than talk however, it is interaction with the feeling of ideal thoughts. For example, you may wish to feel more alive, more centered, more expansive and integrated. The following are very simple statements you can make to yourself in order to enhance feelings of health, but these have to be more than words; these are statements that must be felt in your innermost being in order for their effect to work. Postive thought works through emotion to affect the body. Of course, a core assumption is made here that we are more than what we can see. We are multidimensional beings—call us "spiritual beings in human form." We have a mind that is beyond the physical. This mind, as we have seen in this book, can determine our health.

As you begin to read these affirmations, calm yourself. Take a few slow, deep breaths. Allow the peaceful, healing energy of relaxation to be in your body, allow a feeling of health (of wholeness). Allow the peaceful, healing energy to course through your muscles from head to toe. Allow yourself the luxury of a few seconds, minutes or hours of intentional relaxation. Say—and feel— the following quietly within yourself.

Self Love

I allow love for myself.
I allow the feeling of love.
As I love myself my frequencies raise, and love
    of others becomes simple.
I feel the self love change me.
I feel joy. I allow the joy. I deserve the joy.
When I am joyful, others benefit from my joy.
A happier me resonates and helps others feel
    happy.
I allow love of self. I feel the health of self-love.

Wholeness

I am and therefore am a part of the whole.
I am the whole.
I allow and feel this wholeness of myself and of
    all.
 I feel the health of wholeness.

The Body

I acknowledge my body to be a co-creation of
    the Source of life.

___

I am a powerful being in charge of my body.
I allow my ideal for my body to be felt and
therefore to manifest.
I acknowledge the incredible system of life that
is my body.
I acknowledge the intelligence of the body to
function in many ways that are self-
regulating, without conscious
direction from me.
I love this body.
I allow my great love and respect of this body to
be felt within it.
My love and respect for the body enhances its
health.
My love is a nurturing force for the body.
The more I feel love for the body the more it is
nurtured and the more my ideal size and
shape for my body will be allowed to
manifest.
The more my body is nurtured, the more I am.

Health

Health is everywhere.
I may tap into health at any time.
I may allow health at all times.
I allow health now.
As I allow, I feel the energy of health vibrate
within my whole being.
Health is a frequency of vibration of the highest
order.
I may allow myself the adventure of facilitating

this frequency in my being, of feeling its
    expansiveness.
As I allow more and more the feeling of health,
    I sense the newness and adventure and
    infiniteness of it.
I feel the exhiliration of health.
The feeling is real.
I created this feeling.
I create my feeling state of health and may have
    as much health as I desire.
My desire is the key to my health.

The Mind

There is One Mind or Intelligence.
I am of that Mind.
My mind affects and is affected by that mind.
What I think matters.
All thoughts that have been thought exist.
I may think any thought I wish, including new
    thoughts.
I prefer thoughts that bring me joy.
I prefer thoughts that bring me health.
When I cease to acknowledge anything else, the
    other is the only thing that exists.
This process leads to acknowledgement of the
    one power of Divine Mind.
The destination is the journey.

Give Yourself Health

Part Two:

Health Care Providers
in and Around Seattle and the Eastside

Appendix I:
Health Care Providers

Inclusion of the providers listed in this directory does not imply endorsement either by Turning Point Press, its editors or the authors in this volume, nor does the omission of any provider or clinic imply disapproval.

Counseling

(Section includes: Referral Services, Biofeedback, Career, Clinics, Hypnotherapy, Integrative, Group, Body/Mind Psychotherapy, Nurse, Psychotherapy, Psychology, Religious, Social Work, Stress Management, and Workshops and Seminars.)

REFERRAL SERVICES

Women's Therapy Referral Service. Taking the guesswork out of choosing a therapist since 1976. In-person matching with 3 therapists. 1914 N 34th Street, Suite 206, Seattle, WA 98103-9058, 634-2682.

Health Information Specialist. See listing in "Physicians."

FREE COUNSELING SEARCHES

WE FIND LICENSED COUNSELORS TO FIT YOUR PERSONAL/CAREER NEEDS.
Our services provided in complete privacy and at no cost.
Analysis for your needs include:

CLARITY SEARCH SERVICES INC.
*Location and Fee
*Age and Gender
*Method and Philosophy

You deserve the chance to make the most informed decision possible.
24 Hour Reception/Message Telephone: (206) 547-4029.

BIOFEEDBACK

Rosemary MacGregor, R.N., M.S. Eclectic biofeedback practice includes: proper breathing training, therapeutic imagery, art therapy, self-talk, psychotherapy and hypnosis. Works particularly well for: hypertension, headaches, breathing problems, G.I. troubles, anxiety & pain. Children are welcome. Woodinville, Bellevue and Mt. Vernon offices. 18440 146th Ave. NE, Woodinville, WA 98072 (206) 486-1120.

BODY/MIND PSYCHOTHERAPY

Kathleen A. Higgins, MSW, ACSW. I offer a mind/body approach to healing physical and emotional challenges combining traditional therapy with creative visualization and energy balancing. My speciality is in facilitating people in healing themselves through visualization, meditation and a deeper acceptance of themselves. 6 Lake Bellevue Drive #209, Bellevue, WA 98005, 454-6356.

Nancy Satz, MA, Counseling & bodywork for women. Incest & abuse. ACOA. Co-dependency. Relationships. Recovery from childhood trauma. Grief & loss. Inner child. Family of origin work. Personal growth. Self-esteem. Lesbians. 12 years experience. Mt. Baker area in Seattle. 723-1931.

Symma L. Winston, M.A., MFCC. Counseling the health challenged. All challenges arouse us. Health challenges keep us awake! In a safe and loving atmosphere, find, express and understand the emotions connected with the physical condition. Strengthen your inner spirit and allow your body to respond. I work with individuals, families and groups. Also available for workshops and medical consultation. Eastside office, Bellevue, 746-4716.

Neema Caughran, M.A., LMT, Psychotherapist and Licensed Massage Therapist. Psychotherapy/healing. Creative, in-depth approach combining counseling, art therapy, body awareness. Individual adults, children, families, couples, groups, yoga for large women. In practice since 1976. 2800 East Madison, Seattle, WA 98112 (206) 328-4056.

Center for Movement Arts & Therapy: Stacey Goodrich & Margaret Z. Sutro, Co-Directors. Dedicated to supporting all healing arts invovlving body, movement, emotions and spirit in the quest for personal transformation. Movement therapy sessions for individuals and couples, groups, weekend and intensive workshops, training, support for survivors of sexual abuse. 1100 square foot studio rental. 418 North 35th Street (in Fremont), Seattle, WA 98103-8607, 547-8034.

Reed Svadesh Johnson, M.A., L.M.T., Christine Narayana Hooks, Dipl.-Ing., L.M.T. We invite you for an in-depth exploration of the body-mind-emotional connection through the Orgodynamic$_{sm}$ Approach. Orgodynamics is an energy and body therapy that is a powerful and effective approach to being fully alive, vibrating and pulsating with existence. It goes beyond problems to a place where your own inner knowing and wisdom emerges. 15832 34th Ave NE, Seattle 98155, 361-4700

Eastlake Counseling Group. See listing in "Psychotherapy."

Forras and McDonald Associates, Agnes J. Forras CMHC, MFT; S. John McDonald, M.A., CMHC, MFT. Comprehensive Psychotherapy, Education and Consulting Services. Private practice of Individual, Couple, Family & Group Therapy. Forty years of combined professional experience providing mind/body care. Collaboration with local and national experts in medicine, psychiatry, psychology and the neurosciences as well as theology.

Unique features: Comprehensive assessment to include the biological, psychological, spiritual, social & environmental viewpoints. Psychosocial, psychobiologic, & psycho-neuro-immunologic methodology. Multilevel therapeutic involvement including individual, couple, family & group therapy & weekend intensives as well as discussion groups, seminars, classes & many social activities. A strong social support network, i.e., "buddy system," as a fundamental aspect of care. 10756 Exeter Ave., NE, Seattle, 98125 (206) 367-0756.

CAREER COUNSELING

Christine Cave, M.S.W., NCC. Ready for a Career Change? Find the best fit through career testing (Strong-Campbell,

Myers-Briggs), personal exploration exercises and assessment. Job search, interviewing, and resume skills. 6850 35th NE, Seattle, 98115, 522-0207.

Scott Miners, C.H.C. Career repositioning, enhancement of present career, expanding creativity and accessing intuition and individual creativity in profession, career search or change. Hypnotherapy. Bellevue, Issaquah, 443-5642.

CENTERS & CLINICS

Dan O'Connell, Ph.D., and colleagues. We are a group practice in Mental Health attempting to integrate the strengths of traditional Psychology, Psychiatry and Social Work with a respect for the healing power of one's values and beliefs. We work with all ages and problems utilizing a broad range of approaches. We practice at four locations in and around Seattle and are insurance reimbursable. Mental Health Services, Pacific Medical Center, 1200 12th Ave South, Seattle 98144, 326-4045.

CenteringPoint Clinic. See listing in "Psychotherapy."

GAY & LESBIAN PSYCHOTHERAPY

Eastlake Counseling Group. See listing in "Psychotherapy."

GROUP

InnerLinks Inc., The Transformation Game®. Joy Drake or Kathy Tyler. Consulting, Facilitator Trainings and Seminars. The Transformation Game® is an innovative and dynamic instrument designed to encourage the process of self-discovery, fulfillment of individual and group objectives and creation of new action plans. InnerLinks, P.O. Box 16225, Seattle, WA 98116 (206) 937-0783.

See Bellevue Health & Training, "Education" section.

See Forras McDonald, Body/Mind, this section.

See Jordan-Roberts Sammons, Workshops, this section.

HYPNOTHERAPY

Kavya Kendall, Ericksonian Hypnosis, NLP, Facticity™, 646 32nd Ave E., Seattle, 98112, 325-6565.

L.J. DeHerrera, Ed.D., ABMP, medical psychotherapist-counselor-hypnotherapist. Fellow & Diplomate, American Board of Medical Psychotherapists. Sports Hypnosis-psychotherapy-hypnotherapy-counseling. Adult issues-human development. Emphasis on healing the source, not just the symptom. 2534 125th Av NE, Bellevue, WA 98005, 454-4273.

Merrily Diop, M.H. Besides weight normalization, stopping smoking/drugs/alcohol, ACOA and phobias, I do imagery healing involving self-love and forgiveness. I teach self-hypnosis to every client. I also teach self-esteem imagery classes at Shoreline and Edmonds Community Colleges. 420 Fifth Avenue South. Edmonds 98020 (206) 774-5916.

Innersource, Linda Baker, R.N., C.H.T. & Jennifer Noia, C.H.T. Seek your answers from within—open the doorway to your subconscious mind using: Alchemical (inner-transformational) hypnotherapy; Reiki (Japanese Art of gentle touch therapy) and the work of Louise Hay for: abuse issues, codependency, stop smoking, weight loss, physical challenges, releasing old, unwanted patterns, abortion issues, past life & spiritual awareness, individual sessions, groups, classes. Please call for free brochure & information. 229 Broadway E., Suite 4, Seattle, 322-1055.

Ron Slosky, Ph.D. See listing in "Psychology," this section.

INTEGRATIVE

Laurie A. Dawson, M.A. Working with a transpersonal, eclectic approach to life events, transitions & challenges. Healing, growth & increased personal joy are facilitated. P.O. Box 31593, Seattle, WA 98103 (206) 527-7984, 820-6312.

Alex Gerber, Ph.D. Holistic educator and counselor. P.O. Box 2997, Kirkland, WA 98083, 827-8088.

Pat Stapleton, M.A. Working with you to find and transcend the patterns that are self-destructive and keep you from being fully alive. North Capitol Hill, Seattle (206) 525-1097.

Joanne Dunn, M.A. Synthesis. Loss and growth—counseling and workshops. Box 27181, Seattle, WA 98125, 363-3194.

Forras & McDonald Associates. See listing in "Body/Mind," this section.

MARRIAGE & FAMILY

CenteringPoint Clinic. See listing in "Psychotherapy."

Family Services
serving residents since 1892

461-3883   a United Way agency

Bereavment Services	246-6142
Cancer Lifeline	461-4542
help for those living with cancer	Toll free: 1-800-255-5505
Evergreen Stroke Association/ARISE	461-7839
help for those living with stroke	
Facing Aging Concerns Together	461-3883
meeting the needs of older people & their adult children	
Family Anger Management Institute	461-3883
Family Life Education	461-3883
classes designed to build family skills	
Men Working Against Abuse	461-7824
support for formerly abusive men	

Family Counseling Services:

Bellevue	451-2869	Rainier Valley	461-3880
Greenlake	461-3870	Renton	226-1253
Kent	854-8705	Seattle	461-3883

NURSE

Eastlake Counseling Group. See listing in "Psychotherapy."

Marcella Hunter, R.N. Thoughts develop into beliefs. Beliefs develop into attitudes. Attitudes develop into emotional states. Emotinal climates of long-consistent duration crystalize & impact physiological & physical function. Rebirthing clears stagnant energy from body & mind & allows safe emotional release & relaxation therby re-establishing alignment via the connected breath. I have been a nurse & holistic practitioner for 18 years. My practice is spiritually based. P.O. Box 27712, Seattle, WA 98125-2712 (206) 525-4665.

OLDER ADULTS

Eastlake Counseling Group. See listing in "Psychotherapy."

PSYCHOTHERAPY

Arinna Moon, M.A. Heal your inner self. Grief and loss, depression, abuse, incest, ACOA, medical issues. 6869 Woodlawn Ave., NE, Suite 200, Seattle, 98115, 344-6449.

Lynn Fuller, M.A., M.F.C.C. I offer in-depth psychotherapy from a Jungian perspective for individuals and couples. Authentic movement with individuals and groups is also offered. 4096 Lytle Rd. NE, Seattle, WA 98110, 842-3334.

Healing Choices, Lynda Zahava, M.Ed., LMP (Certified Mental Health Counselor.) Offering effective, individual and group counseling for women seeking freedom from complulsive behaviors, (eating, spending, co-dependency, procrastinating, over-scheduling etc.) Also offering healing massage for men and women. 743 N. 35th, Seattle 98103, 548-9072.

Eleanor Soto, MSW, ACSW, Psychotherapist/consultant, first consultation free. Relationships, ACOA, substance abuse, abuse/incest issues, depression, intercultural conflicts, groups, individual, couples, 16 years experience, Ballard/Phinney Ridge area, 789-5343.

CenteringPoint Clinic, a Team of Counselors and Consultants, committed to the balance of Mind-Body-Emotions-Spirit. Call Co-directors Penny Herman, MA or Robert A. Carlson, MSW. 111 103rd Ave NE, Bellevue, 454-1787.

Simpson & Hare Associates: June Simpson, M.Ed., SCMHC; Patricia Hare, M.Ed., NCC. We specialize in Addictive Relationships, and for the person who loves too much, we offer an assessment to help you evaluate whether to stay or leave a painful relationship. Brochure available. 222 Etruria, Suite 120, Seattle, 98109, 285-1630.

Janet Edlefsen, M.S. My focus is on problems of chronic dieting, preoccupation with food/weight, compulsive eating and bulimia. I help people to make peace with food and their bodies, and achieve normal eating and weight without dieting. I offer individual and group counseling and lectures. 4026 NE 55th, Suite E-241, Seattle, 98105, 524-9496.

Kate R. Casey, M.C., C.D.C. I work with individuals of all ages in individual, couples, family and group settings. I offer an integrated approach that includes; education, experiential process, corrective parenting and spiritual transformation for people recovering from addictions, childhood trauma, transitional stress and other life challenges. 11033 NE 12th, Bellevue, WA 98004, 455-1034.

Carol C. Peters, M.C., N.C.C. I provide both in-depth therapy and brief problem solving therapy for men and women, individually and in groups. I specialize in adult children of alcoholic issues, recovery from childhood incest and sexual abuse, healing the wounded child within, and treating depression. I support clients in developing skills to increase self-esteem, act assertively, move through grieving, create healthy relationships, and confidently direct their lives. Washington State Certified. Evening appointments available. 222 Etruria, Suite 120, Seattle, WA 98109, 282-2180.

Andrea Gamache, Ph.D. Utilizing the body's wisdom and the creative power of thought to generate new possibilities and master life's challenges. Specializing in Chronic Fatigue Syndrome. Adults and children. 10655 NE 4th, Suite 443, Bellevue 98004, 562-1533.

Patricia Wampler, Licensed Counselor. I provide individual and group peer-support counseling based upon using our creativity for negotiating major life changes and important relationships. Call me if you are committed to getting well or improving your life. Over the past 21 years I have helped numerous people work through trauma, addiction and depression. My speciality is chronic distress or patterns which repeat themselves year after year until they are healed. 14306 NE 7th Place, #2, Bellevue 98007 (206) 641-8411.

Shana London, M.C. Gestalt/transformational psychotherapy and the healing art of Jin Shin Jyutsu in a peaceful, wooded setting. Jin Shin Healing Arts, Eastside, 391-0419.

Forras & McDonald Associates. See listing in "Body/Mind," this section.

Leslie D. Schwartz, M.A. Counselor and teacher in psychology and nutrition. 6851 Yacht Haven Road, Friday Harbor, WA 98250 (206) 378-3688.

Carole Milan Danis, MSW ACSW. Twenty years' experience. I am especially effective in assisting adult children to heal from the past, get free of depression, anxiety or compulsive behaviors and create an identity of their own choosing, one that is more satisfying and open to life. My own recovery work provides additional understanding and sensitivity. 1914 N. 34th St., Suite 406, Seattle 98103, 633-0101.

Ron Slosky, Ph.D. See listing in "Psychology," this section.

EASTLAKE COUNSELING GROUP

Feminist-Oriented Psychotherapy for Women and Men

• Elizabeth (Betty) Davisson, ACSW, BCD
• Linda Luster, MD, Child and Adult Psychiatry
• Karen MacQuivey, ACSW, BCD
• Ilene Stein, RN, ACSW

Queen Anne Square, 200 W. Mercer, Suite E-114, Seattle, WA 98119, (206) 361-2465

Sue M. Stevens, MSW, Normandy Park Counseling. Focus on Women's issues, sexuality, couples counseling. 19829 1st Ave So., Seattle 98148 (206) 243-5464 (Tacoma 752-5819).

Doniella Boaz, Psychotherapist, founder of Discoveries workshops and seminars. Her enthusiasm, humor and insight create a safe atmosphere which empowers people to discover and explore their inner world of thoughts and feelings: to nurture and heal their inner Child-Self: to address issues of self-esteem, intimacy, relationship, sexuality, communication. Gorsvenor House, 500 Wall Street, Suite 309, Seattle, WA 98121 (206) 443-5433 or 362-4196.

PSYCHOLOGY

Ron Weiss, Ph.D. I like to work with people who are ready to explore and move through the deeper issues and emotions which underly their current problems. The Process of Integration, which is based on my own experiences in therapy, is the most powerful tool I know for doing this.

The Process of Integration is an intensive, structured program of emotional, intellectual and spiritual development. Beginning with the internal conflict between intellect and emotions as it manifests in guilt, depression, self-indulgence, perfectionism, and the vast array of self-defeating patterns

---

123

and negative emotions, The Process moves toward a penetrating examination of the origins of this conflict. It takes us back to the painful incidents and negative conditioning of our childhood and moves through the pain and anger associated with these events to a new level of clarity and compassion. This makes possible a deeper sense of inner harmony and integration and helps open us to the transpersonal and spiritual dimensions of our being. 2531 152nd Avenue NE, Redmond 98052, 881-3358.

Marian H. Mowatt, Ph.D. Individual and couple psychotherapy, including problems of older adults. Psychological evaluations. 1107 NE 45th St., Suite 405, Seattle 98105, 547-1706.

Kay Roberts McCarthy, Ph.D. Personal or Relationship Stress; Sexuality; Adult Survivors of Childhood Abuse; ACOA. 2105 112th NE, Bellevue, 98004, 451-9191.

John R. Hellman, Ph.D. 515 Minor Avenue, Suite 300, Seattle 98104, 386-9610.

David J. Kosins, Ph.D. Licensed Psychologist, Cognitive Therapy. Treatment of depression, stress, anxiety, panic attacks, & phobias. Individuals-couples-groups. Insurance welcome. 1001 Broadway, Ste. 315, Seattle 98122, 323-0905.

Paul W. Johnson, Ph.D. Licensed psychologist. Queen Anne Psychological Group. Geriatrics specialist. Depression, stress, anxiety. 22 W. Lee, Seattle 98119, 281-7381.

Glenda T. Berg, Ph.D. Spiritual psychology. Queen Anne Psychological Group. 22 W. Lee, Seattle 98119, 281-7381.

Bellevue Psychology Clinic, Drs. DeWitt, Lawson, Ruddell, Anderson,& Slater. 2025 112th Ave NE, # 200, Bellevue 98004, 454-0800.

Saul Breit, Ph.D. Individual psychotherapy, Sexual issues,

Marital & Relationship Issues, Eating Disorders. Insurance eligible. For information. 1899 116th NE, Bellevue, 454-5341.

Mitra Deneuve Seraji, has a Ph.D. in Clinical Psychology with a special interest in treating depression & is currently in private practice. She is also a Fashion & Cosmetic consultant. Lloyd Building, Suite 912, Seattle 98101, 340-0958.

Peter Thomas, Ph.D. Licensed Clinical Psychologist. I work with Process-oriented Psychology & the connections among words, movements, body feelings & symptoms, dreams, relationship problems, & group processes. Insurance eligible. 4649 Sunnyside Ave N, Room 341, Seattle 98103, 547-6772.

Dan O'Connell, Ph.D. See listing in "Clinics."

RELIGIOUS/SPIRITUAL
George C. Fowler, M.A. I assist clients to reassess consciously & critically their self- and God-concepts in light of the human race's store of mystical experience & data. Simultaneously I guide them in meditation to gain their own inner experience of Self & Being. Healing follows spontaneously. 1380 156th NE, #140, Bellevue, 98007, 644-7085.

Genjo Marinello, Zen Priest, C.S.D. I offer a form of consultation called Spiritual Direction, appropriate for anyone seeking to illuminate their Inner-Light, explore & stretch. Kokoro Consulting, 747 16th Ave. E., Seattle, 98112, 328-3944.

SELF-ESTEEM
Heidi E. Burke, MSW, ACSW. 13 years counseling experience with individuals and couples. No charge for 15 minute exploratory consultation. 1400 112th Ave SE, Suite 218, Bellevue 98004, 455-3760.

SOCIAL WORK
Sharon J. Nations, ACSW—Certified Social Worker. Coun-

seling with warmth and challenge for individuals, couples, families with issues about communication, career change, life transitions and emotional well being. I specialize in work with adults from dysfunctional family backgrounds on healing the effects of addiction, abuse or neglect. 2220 Queen Anne Avenue North, Seattle 98109, 284-7922.

Heather J. Chambers, MSW, BCD. 10 years' private practice. Relationships, communication, self-esteem, specialize in survivors of child sexual abuse. 1197 112th NE, #5, Bellevue 98004, 462-9262.

Pam Williamson, MSW, ACSW, Adolescent, Child, and Adult counseling. Psychiatric Social Worker. We all have within us the answers to our own questions and problems. Therapy is a process that aids our quest for those answers. My role as a therapist is to help you find your answers and therefore find balance in your life.

I specialize with adolescents and children, but I see adults as well. I do couple, family and individual therapy with many problem areas. 6353 84th Ave SE, Mercer Island, WA 98040, 232-8333 & 30640 Pacific Hwy S., Federal Way, 98003, 839-1178.

STRESS

Ron Slosky, Ph.D. See listing in "Psychology."

Relax & Live, Inc., Stress Management and self-esteem development; the foundation of programs offered. Private therapy, cassette tapes and group presentations available. Judith Senecal Hoff, president, Jo Ann Abrams, therapist, 4208 198th St. SW, Suite 112, Lynnwood 778-7881.

WORKSHOPS/SEMINARS

Jordan Roberts-Sammons, M.Div. My workshop clients decide their own fees. HOMECOMINGS! provides effective, supportive, workshops as well as individual, couple, & group therapy on dysfunctional family, relationship & self-esteem issues in the warmth & beauty of my 1901 private home. I also offer a rare resource to those who have lost people to suicide. I facilitate your making peace with your past, experiencing joy in the present, and having confidence in the future. Squire Park, 718 16th Avenue, Seattle 98122, 329-7616.

Forras & McDonald Associates. Comprehensive Psychotherapy, Education & Consulting Services. Monthly psychospiritual retreats dedicated to offering the experience of Unconditional Love, Forgiveness, & Gratitude. Seminars on Marriage Enrichment, Sacred Sexuality, Life Purpose & Values, & Growth through Completion & Redecision. See full description in Counseling (Body/Mind Psychotherapy). 367-0756.

Dental

Mitch Marder, D.D.S. In our dental practice, one receives the highest quality dental care available in a warm, caring & friendly atmosphere. We offer mercury free dentistry, appropriate referral for metal-toxicity screening, & nutritional approaches to periodontal health. We are comfortable working with herbal & homeopathic alternative medications. We believe dental health is intimately related to whole body health; including physical, mental, emotional, behavioral & environmental factors. 822 A, NE Northgate Way, Seattle, 98125, 367-6453.

John August Rau, D.D.S., M.A. Mercury-free Restorative Dentistry, emphasizing gold & ceramics. Nutritional approach to Periodontal Disease. Huggins protocol available. Brochure available. 1328 Medical-Dental Building, Seattle 98101 (206) 622-2380

ADAMS (A Dental Amalgam Mercury Syndrome). ADAMS is a non-profit organization formed by persons recovering from various illnesses which M.D.s have linked to an intolerance of the material in their dental fillings. ADAMS provides public education through the role of books, pamphlets, and video-tapes. Also provided is patient support through monthly meetings and quarterly newsletters. ADAMS is open to membership from the general public. Write or phone, P.O. Box 854, Kirkland, WA 98083-0854, 822-2765.

Education & Schools

(Section includes: Bach Remedial Training, Counseling & Hypnosis, Massage Therapy Training, Rebirthing & Relationships Training.)

BACH REMEDIAL TRAINING

Dee Hall, M.A. Seattle's only certified Bach Flower consultant/teacher. Registered with Bach Centres USA and Oxfordshire, England. Consultations, Lecutres, Workshops.

Used as directed, Bach Flower Remedies can alleviate a wide range of mental & emotional stresses. Uscd worldwide for 1/2 century! 4411 4th Av. NE, Seattle 98105, 633-2117.

COUNSELING AND HYPNOSIS

Inner Links Inc., The Transformation Game® (See "Group" in Counseling section.

Institute for Re-Education of the Unconscious Mind (I.R.E.U.M.)—certification in Ericksonian Hypnosis, NLP and Facticity. IREUM is a Washington State approved private vocational school. Trainings emphasize developing the creativity, flexibility & conscious awareness of the health care practitioner. Ragini Elizabeth Michaels, Director and Main Trainer. Contact: P.O. Box 22814, Seattle 98122, 462-4369.

MASSAGE TRAINING PROGRAMS

The Brenneke School of Massage provides excellence in

massage therapy training. We teach from both the clinical and holistic viewpoints and bring to our students a combined seventy years of professional experience.

•The Brenneke School's acclaimed 550-hour **Professional Massage Licensing Program** prepares the student for the Washington State Board Examinations and a career in massage therapy.

•**Advanced Training Seminars** present specialized techniques designed to broaden the health-care provider's skills and treatment capabilities: Integrative Deep Tissue, Connective Tissue, On-Site, and Sports Massage; AIDS Training; Polarity Balancing; Shiatsu; Autogenic Training; Ortho-Bionomy™, and Foot Reflexology.
•And we offer fun and challenging **workshops for the nonprofessional.** Brenneke School of Massage . . . providing excellence in Massage Therapy Training since 1974. 160 Roy Street, Seattle, WA 98109. 282-1233.

Brian Utting School of Massage. 900 Thomas St., Seattle, Washington, 98109 (206) 292-8055.

Bellevue Health & Training Center is a small, certified 650-hour massage training school that provides a student clinic. Class maximum of eight students insures individualized attention. Call for information about additional specialized mini-courses. Student clinic massage therapy, open to the public, $15-pregnant women welcome. *(**Counseling**: Groups for sexual abuse) also other services/products.

REBIRTHING & RELATIONSHIPS
The Loving Relationships Training (LRT) is a psychological and spiritual study of how your past affects your present relationships. It offers amazing tools to resolve barriers and manifest anything you want. By the end of the LRT you won't be able to pretend you don't know what's going on any more. For more information call us or read Sondra Ray's and Bob

Mandel's books. P.O. Box 1928, Woodinville, WA 98072 (206) 481-5270.

Healing Arts

(Section includes: Breath Therapy, Chiropractic, Health Counseling, Healing Touch, Licensed Massage Therapists— acupressure, cranio-sacral, Heller, Neuro-muscular, Reflexology, Rolfing, Shiatsu, Swedish, Trager.)

BREATH THERAPY

Rebirthing is a powerful method of healing and personal growth which uses the breath to release stress & supressed emotions, thus making it possible to experience more joy and aliveness. •Tim Barlen, LRT Sponsored Rebirther, 923 E. John St., Apt. 303, Seattle, 98102, 329-4344. •Joan Dacres, LRT Sponsored Rebirther, 629 NW 82nd St., Seattle, 98117, 783-7354. •Cindy McDonell, LRT Sponsored Rebirther, 7522 10th Ave NW, Seattle, 98117, 789-5145. •Sharon Nations, M.S.W., 2220 Queen Anne Ave. N., Seattle, 98109, 284-7922.

Marcella Hunter, R.N. See listing in Counseling (Nurse).

Peter and Meg Kane, The LRT. See listing in Education (Rebirthing and Relationships Training)

COLON THERAPY

Healthworks. Colon Therapy Specialists. Are you experiencing gas, bloating, constipation, fatigue, indigestion, headaches, bad breath? The health of the colon can have wideranging effects on the rest of the body, mind & spirit. Cleansing the colon can relieve these symptoms as well as facilitate clarity of thought & a higher sense of well-being. We use the Wood's Gravity Flow System which involves gentle irrigation with purified water & implants (wheatgrass, aloe, minerals and healthy bacteria) to eliminate toxins, restore normal flora

& maintain healthy bowel function. Individualized cleansing programs suited to your needs & goals. Beautiful environment. Products. books. Affiliated with N.D., D.C., M.D., O.M.D., C.A. LMPs certified in Colon Therapy. 2719 E. Madison, Suite 302, Seattle 98112, 726-8568.

Bellevue Health & Training. See listing in "Education"

DANCE/MOVEMENT THERAPY

Center for Movement Arts & Therapy. See lising in Counseling (Body/Mind Psychotherapy).

HEALTH CENTERS

Khalsa Health Center. Holistic clinic, herbology specialists—allergy (food, inhalant), virus, chronic fatigue. 1305 NE 45th St., Suite 205, Seattle, 98105, 547-2007.

Northwest Center for Attitudinal Healing, Adults with life-threatening or chronic illness-support groups. Contact person: Patty Hesslin, 11700 1st Ave NE, Seattle, 98125, 782-5530.

HEALING TOUCH

Kandy B. Brandt, Reiki Master. Channelling Reiki, universal life energy, accelerates the body's ability to heal physical ailments, opens the mind and spirit to the causes of disease and pain, and restores balanced aliveness. 2609 Broadway East, Seattle, 98102, 328-6065.

Shana London, M.D. Jin Shin Jyutsu. See (Psychotherapy).

HEALTH COUNSELING

Symma L. Winston, M.A., M.F.C.C. Counseling the health challenged. With any health challenge there are emotional components, needing to be expressed, understood and used for accessing the vital force we need to regain our wholeness. My work is guiding individuals, families and groups to their own inner resources. I am also available for workshops and medical consultations. Eastside office, Bellevue, 746-4716.

LICENSED MASSAGE THERAPISTS

Inspired Bodywork. Structural, Polarity and Cranial Balancing for optimum health and well-being. Therapeutic massage using deep and subtle tissue techniques. I work with stress responses and emotional content, tension patterns and structural compensation, body alilgnment and energetic balance. Brochure available. Roosevelt District, Seattle. By appointment: 523-1093

Bellevue Health & Training. See listing in "Education."

The Brenneke School of Massage, Health & Treatment Center features: Swedish massage therapy for stress release and relaxation; and Sports massage and deep tissue treatment for athletes and others with musculoskeletal conditions. 160 Roy Street, Seattle, 98109, 282-1233.

Therapeutic Massage Clinic, Kari Elliott, L.M.T., L.C. Using methods including Swedish, Positional Release, Neuro-Muscular Re-education, Reflexology, OrthoBionomy™, and Polarity, we work to release patterns of stress. Programs for weight control, fitness and flexibility. Specializing in chronic pain relief and post trauma therapy. 10116 Main Street, Suite 104, Bothell, WA 98011, 486-0457.

Chris Pringer, L.M.T. Integrative Bodywork goes in-depth with the tissues to clarify and release the issues; increases the interconnectedness of the body and mind. Highly trained and experienced. 1508 35th Ave., Seattle, 98122, 324-6980.
Bettelinn, L.M.T. Ashtanga Yoga, Therapeutic Massage, Jin Shin Jyutsu Acupressure, Foot Reflexology. 363-5517.

Daisie Kallop, L.M.T. Serving Seattle 17 years. Great massage treatments, reflexology, Chinese ear wax removal, and rebirthing. Classes available. Call 547-3866.

Jo Roalkvam, L.M.T. Is your life filled with stress? Try therapeutic massage. Swedish and Deep Muscle. 643-4819.

Lakeside Massage Clinic, "The Injury Clinic." 7300 E. Greenlake Dr. N., Seattle 98115.

Lynwood Oriental Healing Arts Clinic. Carol Conlon, C.A. and Dan Chaffee, L.M.P. offer body "tune-ups" that both relax and help restore your self-healing response. Helps pain, addictions, internal organ disease, immune system and muscular-skeletal problems. Our healing methods are always safe, effective and gentle. 20102 Cedar Valley Road, Lynnwood, WA 98036, 776-5353.

Julia Heneghan, L.M.P. I have been a practicing massage therapist for twenty years. I specialize in Swedish massage for reducing stress, Sports massage for athletic type injuries and other techniques for those suffering from chronic illness. 3876 Bridgeway N., Suite 202, Seattle 98103, 547-8382.

Rex Holt, Certified Rolfer. Rolfing is for people who want improved posture, athletic performance, increased body-awareness and energy and body comfort. Free consultations. 14655 Bel-Red Rd., Ste 105, Bellevue, Wash., 98007, 747-5246.

Nancy Satz, M.A. Hawaiin/emotional release bodywork. 723-1931.

Swedish, Sports & Therapeutic Massage Clinic, Katherine Cantrell, owner. 1402 3rd Ave, Seattle 98101 623-1391.

Alan Kaplan, Certified Rolfer. Rolfing is a process of change; I work with clients to realize physical and emotional goals through evoking balance and integration in the body. 4332 Meridian Ave. N., Seattle, 98103, 548-9165.

Barbara Jacobsen, Certified Rolfer. The woman Rolfer on the Eastside. 413 14th Ave W., Kirkland, 98033, 822-6433, Seattle, 522-2595.

Beth Cachat, Certified Trager^R Practitioner, L.M.P., 7205 NE 156th, Bothell, WA 98011, 488-1470.

Reed Svadesh Johnson, M.A. and Christine Narayana-Hooks, Dipl. Ing., Trager^R. 15832 34th Ave NE, Seattle, 98155, 361-4700.

Yasuo Mori, Japanese Shiatsu Therapy. Sorrento Hotel, 900 Madison Street, Seattle, 464-0757.

Janine Powell, R.N., L.M.P. Relaxing Swedish massage. Gift certificates. N. Seattle, 367-2518.

Inspired Bodywork. See beginning of this section—craniosacral work.

YOGA

Aadil B.A. Palkhivala, J.D., Director, Iyengar Yoga Institute of Washington State (I.Y.I.W.S.). Iyengar Yoga is the world's most refined and practical yoga system, & the only complete exercise known. Improve your general health, mental, physical or emotional performance.

Aadil has studied with Yoga Master B.K.S. Iyengar for 23 years, holds an advanced teacher's certificate, & is internationally renowned as the teacher of teachers.

Personalized therapeutic, private or all-level classes. Eastside and Seattle. First class free. P.O. Box 70496, Bellevue, WA 98007 (206) 883-7667.

Yoga and Self-Image for large women. Neema Caughran. See listing in Counseling (Body/Mind Psychotherapy).

Movement and Fitness

(Includes: Aikido, Aquarobics, Feldenkrais, T'ai Chi Ch'uan.)

AIKIDO

Pamela Cooper, Chief Instructor, 4th Degree Black Belt. Aikido is Japan's modern nonviolent martial art. Aikido brings together the mind, body and spirit into one harmonious force. Aikido of West Seattle, 4745 40th SW, Suite #206, Seattle, 98116, 938-5222/547-2183.

AQUAROBICS™

Aquarobics™ water exercise by Judy Mills, L.M.P. Mind and body connecting in the safest exercise environment: Aquarobics™ water exercise, solid fitness for your future. 13240 Northup Way, Suite #14, Bellevue 98005, 641-4006.

FELDENKRAIS™

Margaret Graham, MOT, OTR-L. Learn to release tension, increase ease and awareness of movement and posture; classes, individual sessions. Seattle 783-1942.

T'AI CHI CH'UAN

Colleen Donovan, T'ai Chi Instructor, N. Seattle, 633-3561.

Physicians

(Section includes: Referral /Research Services, Acupuncturists, Chiropractic, Clinics, General, Homeopathic, Naturopathic, Optometrist.)

REFERRAL/RESEARCH SERVICES

Janice Guthrie, Health Information Specialist. You can be

135

informed about your medical problem & thoroughly explore your treatment options with an individualized research report on your specific condition. Reports include information on the latest conventional & alternative treatments, nutrition, specialists, more. Write or call: The Health Resource, 209-B, Katherine Drive, Conway, AR 72032 (501) 329-5272.

CHIROPRACTIC

Seattle Chiropractic Health Center. Dr. David Weber. Welcome to the beginning of the end of your pain. Through specific analysis and gentle adjustments we help you get back to sound structural health. Personalized, individual treatment. 2004 Fairview Ave, Seattle, WA 98121 (206) 623-6800.

Richard C. Bartlett, D.C. Discover the natural chiropractic approach to health. Quality individualized care to meet your health and wellness goals. Corrective and preventive care. Medical Dental Bldg., 509 Olive Way, Suite 1342, Seattle, 98101, 467-6479.

CLINICS

Natural Health Clinic of Bastyr College: Mark Bresnick, MSW, MHA, Clinic Director; Dr. Eric Jones, ND, Chief Medical Officer; Drs. Jane Guiltinan, ND, Pam Houghton, ND, John Hibbs, ND, Suzy Adams, ND, Robert Ullman, ND and Maureen O'Keefe, MA Clinical Faculty.

Wellness, naturally. Primary Health Care Services support your body's inherent healing mechanisms with proven therapies. General family practice medical care; women's health care; cervical caps; homeopathy; nutritional consulting; personal counseling; physical medicine. Specialized treatment packages: Quit smoking; lose weight; HIV+/ARC/AIDS. Some insurance coverage, State L&I. 1408 NE 45th, Seattle 98105, 632-0354.

GENERAL

Leo J. Bolles, M.D. Inc. P.S.—Preventive Medicine. My approach is to look for the cause of a problem, and treat it with nutrition and homeopathy first. My emphasis in practice is: •Nutrition and Allergy Testing. •Homeopathic Remedies. •Chelation Therapy. 15611 Bel-Red Rd., Bellevue, WA 98008. Phone (206) 881-2224.

HOMEOPATHIC

Robert M. Schore, M.D. I am a fully qualified family practice physician specializing in classical homeopathic medicine for over fifteen years. My practice includes extensive patient evaluation and requires active patient participation. I find my medical practice rewarding in that it usually leads to healing the underlying causes of illness. This means that patients experience virtual elimination of the possibility of adverse drug reactions and more freedom from susceptibility to chronic disease. My purpose is to help patients achieve and maintain good health and a higher quality of life. 3216 NE 45th Place, Suite 304, Seattle, WA 98105, 525-8722.

Robert Ullman, N.D., D.H.A.N.P. and Judyth Reichenberg-Ullman, N.D., D.H.A.N.P., M.S.W. The Northwest Center for Holistic Medicine, 4072 9th Ave., NE, Seattle, WA 98105, 547-9665 (See listing in "Naturopathic" Physicians.)

NATUROPATHIC

Hope Faith, N.D., L.M. Naturopathic physician and licensed midwife using nutrition and digestive therapy, including colon therapy, stool and parasite testing. Also using botanicals, homeopathy and electromagnetic therapy.

Specializing in natural childbirth and refacilitation of birth trauma in infants and children and women's health issues; including, fitting of diaphragms and cervical caps.

Always working toward a balance between the emotional, spiritual and physical bodies. 8315 5th Ave. NE, Suite A, Seattle, WA 98115 (206) 527-1366.

Robert Ullman, N.D., D. HANP and Judyth Reichenberg-Ullman, N.D., D. HANP, M.S.W. The Northwest center for Holistic Medicine. We specialize in healing body, mind, and spirit and discovering the roots of illness. We use homeopathy, Ayurveda, herbs, nutrition, and transformational counseling and hypnosis. Also available are cervical caps, diaphragms, colon therapy, massage, sauna, and hot tub. We also teach, write, and lecture extensively. 4072 9th Ave. NE, Seattle, WA 98105, 547-9665.

Eastside Naturopathic Clinic. Three Naturopathic Physicians, Two acupuncturists and two midwives have come together, blending Eastern and Western healing traditions. They have created a vision of cooperative holistic medicine for the community, and extend their healing approach to you and your family. 607 Market St., Kirkland, WA 98033 (206) 822-3716.

John Bastyr Clinic. See listing in "Clinics" this section.

OPTOMETRY

Dr. George N. Dever, O.D. and Associates. We offer tradiional and alternative therapies to help you achieve your goals in vision. Individualized programs may include: vision recovery classes, eye exercises, biofeedback, color therapy, nutrition, and counseling.

We work in the areas of prescription reduction, strabismus, amblyopia, visually related learning problems, cataract, glaucoma, macular degeneration, and dry eye. 1511 3rd Ave., Suite 411, Seattle 98101, 634-0737.

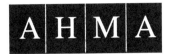

AMERICAN HOLISTIC MEDICAL ASSOCIATION
Physicians dedicated to medicine for the whole person

The American Holistic Medical Association (AHMA) was founded in 1978 to unite fully-licensed physicians who practice holistic medicine. AHMA membership is open to licensed Medical Doctors (M.D.s) Doctors of Osteopathy (D.O.s) and to medical students studying for those degrees. AHMA, a non-profit organization, is involved in educating professionals and the public, advocating insurance coverage of holistic methods, conducting research and broadening public health policies to incorporate preventive and holistic health principles.

American Holistic Medical Foundation
The mission of the American Holistic Medical Foundation (AHMF) is to support research and educational projects promoting holistic medicine.

Fundraising is accomplished through tax-deductible donations, grants and annual AHMF membership fees. Membership in the AHMF is open to all individuals and organizations who share the vision of holistic medicine embodied by AHMA.

The American Holistic Medical Association's national office will furnish a list of physician members by state. The AHMA/AHMF Member Directory includes addresses, phone numbers and specialty information of physicians throughout the United States. It is available for purchase through the national office, as is HOLISTIC MEDICINE, the Associations's bi-monthly journal.

American Holistic Medical Association
4101 Lake Boone Trail, Suite 201
Raleigh, North Carolina 27607   (919) 787-5146

Appendix II:
Health Care Products

Inclusion of the products listed in this directory does not imply endorsement either by Turning Point Press, its editors or the authors in this volume, nor does the omission of any product imply disapproval.

Diet & Food

(Section includes: Herbs, Natural and Organic foods, Supplements and Vitamins.)

HERBS

Gloria DeGaetano, M.E., Independent Distributor, Sunrider International. Sunrider herbs are grown organically and processed with the utmost care and rigorous quality control. The company's philosophy is the ancient Chinese principle of regenerating the body through herb nutrition designed for specific body systems. Sunrider's nutrition and weight management programs incorporate the concentrated herbal formulas the ancients believed would restore balance to the body. I market the products and provide free educational consultations for learning how "to give ourselves optimal health through optimal herb nutrition." 12121 NE 149th St., Kirkland, WA 98034, 488-4595

Arise and Shine Herbal Products. Home of the "Clean-Me-Out Program." Box 99566, Seattle 98199, 286-7634.

SUPPLEMENTS

Light Force. We specialize in state of the art comprehensive nutritional programs for individuals and businesses. We are best known for our medical research with PHYCOTENE™ and our pharmaceutical grade SPIRULINA. Our focus areas include Immune System Building, Peak Performance, Stress Management, and Weight Control. TOLL FREE NATIONWIDE: 1-800-635-4448.

Shaklee Products/in harmony with nature & good health. Sensible supplementation, healthy needs & snacks—backed by clinical research. Jayme Curley, Seattle, 547-8131, Betsy Bell, Seattle 329-6156.

VITAMINS

Great Earth Vitamins. Quality Natural Vitamins at Down to Earth Prices. 221 Bellevue Square, Bellevue 98004.

Bellevue Health & Training. See listing in "Education."

Products & Supplies

(Section includes: Air & Water Purification & Filtration Equipment, Biofeedback & Integration Equipment, Books, Cassette Tapes—audio & video—for Relaxation/health, Environmentally Safe Personal Care, Cleaning & Home Maintenance Products, Lighting, Sexual Health.)

AIR & WATER PURIFICATION

Pure & simple water treatment system. Five stage pressed carbon block system. The only system listed by the National Sanitation Foundation to rcmove lead from your drinking water, as well as pesticides, chemicals, chlorine and organic bacteria. Under-counter or movable units available. 3226 NE 87th, Seattle, 98115, 525-4229, Rick or Cindy.

Flowright Healthful Living Products. See listing in "Environmentally Safe . . . Products & Services" this section.

Pureflow Air Treatment System. A solution to indoor home or office pollution. Reduces smoke, dust or pollen by over 90% in just 30 minutes in a 10x12 foot room. Portable. P.O. Box 15720, Seattle, 98115-0720, 525-4229, Rick or Cindy.

Multi-pure Water Systems. Removes Chemicals, Heavy Metals, Asbestos, Bacteria etc. Complete Ind. lab tests. Portable or under counter units available for pennies per gal. Stainless steel or plastic, both with a 10 yr. warranty. Carbon block, Reverse Osmosis and Shower Systems available. Free in-home trials. Distributor opportunities—full or part-time. No inventory. Independent Distributors: Shirley Wilkinson, Greater Seattle, 524-5642. Donnyl Gunshol, Mercer Is., Bellevue, Kirkland, 236-1783. Phil & Kathy Hayden, Edmonds, Lynnwood, Everett. 776-8089. Don Sanford, Northern Snohomish, Skagit County, La Conner and Bellingham, 466-4651. Lee P. Strenge, South King County, Tacoma area, Pierce County, 752-2838.

H2O—Shaklee Bestwater Purification units. We have 3 filters, including reverse osmosis, removing virtually all types of contaminants. Sales leaders, Betsey Bell, Montlake, 329-6156, Jayme Curley, Wallingford, 547-8131. Distributors: Robin Gruber, Lynnwood, 776-7351. Susan Hartry, N. Seattle, 368-9356. Lynne Jacquay, Redmond, 883-7111. Pamela Knowles, S. Seattle, 722-7282. Ella Mae Kurashige, Bothell, 485-6223. Sue & Eric Landeen, N. Capitol Hill, 329-8636. Cora Lawrence, U. District, 633-3049. Sandy Newell, Wedgewood, 527-2546. Jo Ann Rouga, Renton, 228-5009.

BOOKS & CASSETTE & VIDEO TAPES

Cleanse & Purify Thyself, by Rich Anderson. An easy-to-read and inspiring book on complete intestinal cleansing and digestive rejuvenation with detailed instructions for the "Clean-Me-Out-Program." Includes generous quotes from the Essene Gospel of Peace in which the disciple John gives Jesus' instructions on purifying the Temple. Arise & Shine, P.O. Box 99566, Seattle, 98199 (206) 286-7634.

ENVIRONMENTALLY SAFE PERSONAL, HOME MAINTNANCE & CLEANING CARE

Flowright—Healthful Living Products. Products for the Environmentally Aware, Chemically Sensitive and allergy relief. Non-toxic building and household products; paints, finishes, floor finish, sealants, adhesives, shampoo, laundry &

dish soap etc. AIR: Chemical and or particulate control for the automobile, portable or whole house. Air qulaity testing. WATER: General ecology, Seagull IV, the only product issued a letter of acceptance from the EPA as a "Non-Chemical Purification Device." Stainless housing employs microfiltration (.4 absolute) broad spectrum absorption and electro-kinetic attraction to remove bacteria, chemical pollutants (chlorine, THMs, pesticides) asbestos, etc., while leaving in essential minerals. Portable, point of use & whole house. Water testing. Also rainbow vacuum cleaners, safe space heaters, books, home construction consulting and more. Free brochure or appointment. Retail & wholesale. 1495 NW Gilman Blvd., #4, Issaquah, WA 98027 (206) 392-8357.

LIGHTING

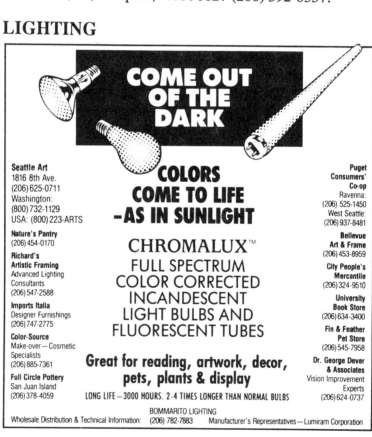

COME OUT OF THE DARK

COLORS COME TO LIFE – AS IN SUNLIGHT

CHROMALUX™

FULL SPECTRUM
COLOR CORRECTED
INCANDESCENT
LIGHT BULBS AND
FLUORESCENT TUBES

Great for reading, artwork, decor, pets, plants & display

LONG LIFE – 3000 HOURS. 2-4 TIMES LONGER THAN NORMAL BULBS

Seattle Art
1816 8th Ave.
(206) 625-0711
Washington:
(800) 732-1129
USA: (800) 223-ARTS

Nature's Pantry
(206) 454-0170

Richard's
Artistic Framing
Advanced Lighting
Consultants
(206) 547-2588

Imports Italia
Designer Furnishings
(206) 747-2775

Color-Source
Make-over — Cosmetic
Specialists
(206) 885-7361

Full Circle Pottery
San Juan Island
(206) 378-4059

Puget
Consumers'
Co-op
Ravenna:
(206) 525-1450
West Seattle:
(206) 937-8481

Bellevue
Art & Frame
(206) 453-8959

City People's
Mercantile
(206) 324-9510

University
Book Store
(206) 634-3400

Fin & Feather
Pet Store
(206) 545-7958

Dr. George Dever
& Associates
Vision Improvement
Experts
(206) 624-0737

BOMMARITO LIGHTING
Wholesale Distribution & Technical Information: (206) 782-7883   Manufacturer's Representatives — Lumiram Corporation

SEXUAL HEALTH RESOURCES

The Rubber Tree. Low cost, non-prescription contraceptives; safe sex supplies. Free referrals, information. Comfortable atmosphere. Mail order available. 4426 Burke Avenue N., Seattle, 98103, 633-4750.